LYM

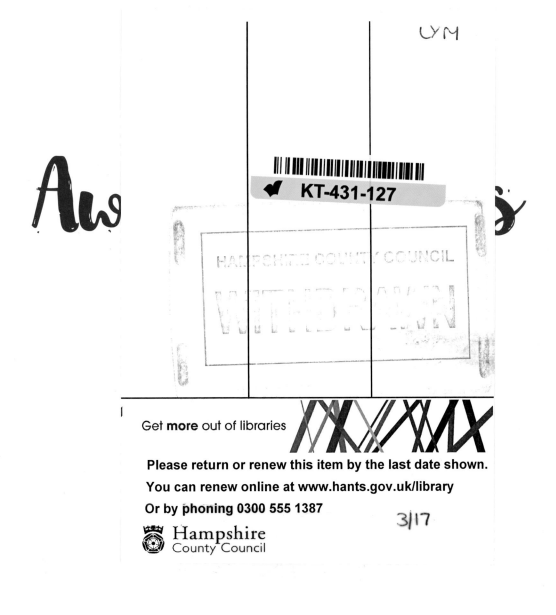

Get **more** out of libraries

Please return or renew this item by the last date shown.

You can renew online at www.hants.gov.uk/library

Or by phoning 0300 555 1387

3/17

Hampshire
County Council

An Hachette UK Company
www.hachette.co.uk

First published in Great Britain in 2017 by Mitchell Beazley,
a division of Octopus Publishing Group Ltd,
Carmelite House, 50 Victoria Embankment,
London, EC4Y 0DZ
www.octopusbooks.co.uk

A CIP catalogue record for this book is available from the
British Library.

ISBN 978-1-78472-283-8

This book was conceived, designed and produced by
RotoVision
Ovest House, 58 West Street,
Brighton, East Sussex
BN1 2RA
United Kingdom

Publisher: Mark Searle
Editorial Director: Isheeta Mustafi
Commissioning Editor: Alison Morris
Editor: Emma Hill
Junior Editor: Abbie Sharman
Art Director: Michelle Rowlandson
Book layout: JC Lanaway
Photographer: Neal Grundy
Cover design: Michelle Rowlandson
Illustrator: Elizaveta Dmitrievna

10 9 8 7 6 5 4 3 2 1

Printed in China by 1010 Printing International Ltd.

Awesome Nails

CREATIVE IDEAS FOR HANDMADE NAIL ART WITH STICKERS, DECALS AND WRAPS

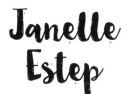

Janelle
Estep

OF ELLEANDISH

MITCHELL
BEAZLEY

CONTENTS

Decal Designs

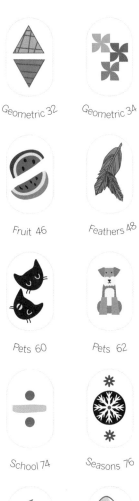 Geometric 32

Geometric 34

 Tribal 36

 Tribal 38

 Food 40

 Food 42

 Fruit 44

Fruit 46

Feathers 48

Feathers 50

Floral 52

 Floral 54

 Ocean 56

Ocean 58

Pets 60

Pets 62

Forest Animals 64

Forest Animals 66

Love 68

  Love 70

School 72

  School 74

Seasons 76

Seasons 78

Pastel Fantasy 80

Pastel Fantasy 82

   Galaxy 84

Galaxy 86

Beauty 88

Beauty 90

Animal Print 92

Animal Print 94

Fashion 96

Fashion 98

Travel 100

 Travel 102

  Music 104

Music 106

 Crystals 108

   Crystals 110

How to use this book

Nail polish was invented thousands of years ago in China as a fashionable status symbol. During the 19th century in Europe and the United States, coloured nail polish salons became popular among the general public. Today, painting your nails and creating nail art is a fun form of personal artistic expression. Nail trends vary from simple French manicures and petite floral designs all the way through to wild nail art themes and explosions of iridescent colours and glitter.

I have been painting my nails since I was a young girl. Growing up, I loved art and I remember being entranced by the world of colour in school supplies such as markers, crayons and coloured pencils. As I got older, I taught myself how to paint my fingernails and toenails and after I finished university I used books and the Internet to teach myself how to edit videos. I uploaded my first nail art tutorial on YouTube in 2012 and my nail art channel has grown in leaps and bounds ever since. I love nail art and nail polish because having beautiful nails is achievable for everyone and will never go out of style. This book teaches you how to beautify your nails with decals. Use the templates supplied and design your own from scratch with printable waterslide decal paper.

Decide what to wear
In Chapter 1 we will look for inspiration and decide what decals you want to wear:

- Explore textile designs, photographs, stills from your favourite films, magazines, newspapers or stationery, or be inspired by nature.
- Go wild with your imagination and have fun choosing subjects that appeal to you.
- Pull together various design elements that you love and plan out a manicure that is truly your own.
- Map out your mani by deciding on your designs for each nail and measure your nail-bed dimensions for a perfect fit.

Create your decals
In Chapter 2 you will find out everything you need to know to draw and design your own nail decals:

- Create your own designs with a computer, or draw them freehand and scan them to resize.
- Learn how to manipulate images with design software, and print them onto your own decal paper to create custom nail decals.
- Step-by-step instructions will then guide you through applying the nail decals, and tips are provided on how to make them last.

Get inspired
Chapter 3 is filled with inspirational decal ideas for your next manicure, from cupcakes and kitty designs to geometrics and zebra print patterns. Use the QR codes on each of the decal pages to download the designs or use the templates on page 28 to create your own bespoke decals. The freestyle tips and thumbnail images found alongside the decal designs reflect the techniques in the photographs, helping you to accurately recreate the featured manicures.

Customize your decals
In Chapter 4 you will learn how to embellish your nail decals with fun decorations! Colour in your decals with nail polish and glitter for a personalized look.

Take care of your nails
Nail art is a form of personal self-expression, so it's important to give your nails the proper care they deserve. In Chapter 5 you will learn:

- The best practices for cuticle care.
- How to file your nails into the three most popular nail shapes.
- DIY tips for a perfect at-home manicure.

Are you ready to beautify your nails with customized nail decals? Let's get started!

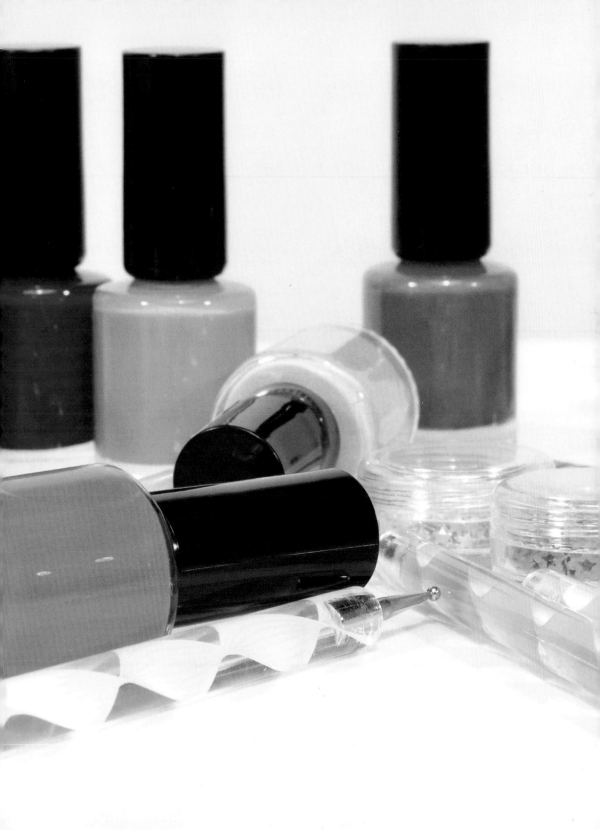

1 WHAT DO YOU WANT TO WEAR?

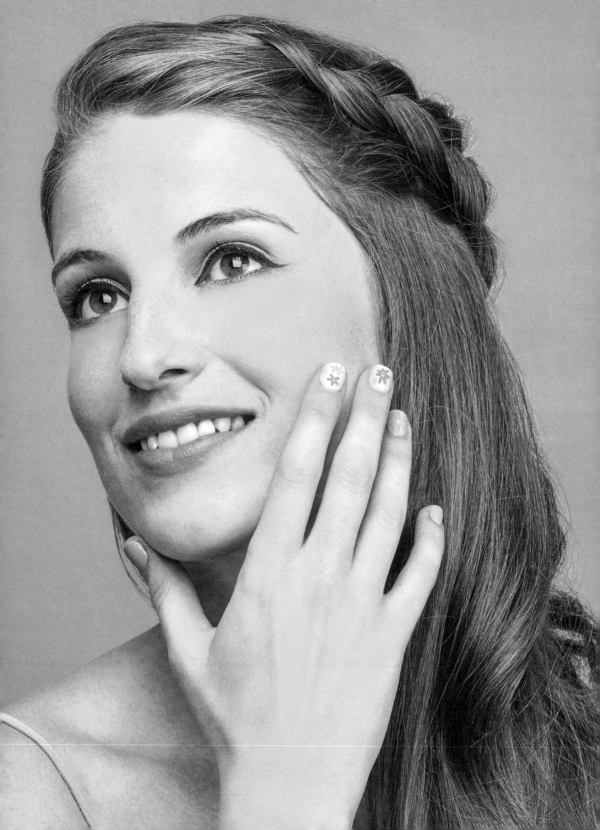

What are nail decals?

If you have ever wanted beautiful and intricate nail designs without spending hours doing them yourself or having to pay someone to paint them on for you, you can apply nail decals! You can use the designs straight out of this book, customize them or create your own.

Temporary tattoos for your nails

Update your nail designs whenever you like with a single polish change, without the hassle of painting designs freehand. Water-transfer nail decals are quick and easy to apply, and unique! You can add any decal to your existing manicure – think of them as temporary tattoos for your nails. Waterslide nail decals can be used with natural, false, acrylic and gel nails. After sealing with a topcoat, nail decals stay on for days. They are durable and long-lasting. . . at least until you decide to update your manicure! Release the decals from the backing paper using water and apply them for an instant accent to your manicure.

Choose decal designs straight from this book, or make your own from scratch (refer to Chapter 2). Let your imagination run wild and create beautiful nail decal designs.

Embellishing your decals

Apply decorations on top of your decals to create three-dimensional art that really pops! Use ordinary nail topcoat, or nail glue for a stronger hold (see page 118). The most popular embellishments are:

• Studs: These are usually made out of metal or plastic – simple geometric shapes are very popular. They can have various colours and finishes.

• Rhinestones: These are typically found as round, flat-backed jewels in glass or plastic. Like nail studs, they come in various sizes, colours and finishes. They can bring bling to an otherwise daytime look.

• Three-dimensional charms and decorations: Nail decorations can be moulded into any shape – flowers, feathers, bows, hearts and more. They can be cast in either plastic or metal.

Alongside your nail decals and embellishments, play with nail colour combos – the possibilities are endless!

Choosing your decals

FIND INSPIRATION

The first step in choosing your nail decals is to decide on a subject. Perhaps you love dogs and you want an adorable puppy-themed nail look. Maybe your favourite festival is approaching and you would like a complementary mani to celebrate the season. If you are still not sure, get inspired! Look at patterns on clothes and in nature, search your favourite magazines for photographs and illustrations, look for themes in films. . . and take note of what resonates with you and fuels your imagination. Have fun with it, because nail art is all about expressing yourself.

Common nail art subjects and themes:
• Festivals
• Seasons
• Florals
• Graphic symbols
• Animals and insects
• Travel destinations
• Food
• Simple text
• Film themes

Once you have settled upon your nail decal subject, gather your inspirational sources together and identify what they have in common to find your manicure style. Write them down to filter out the things that do not fit and pinpoint elements that do:

- Are you drawn to clean lines?
- Do graphic prints catch your eye?
- Do you love bright, all-over colour or subtle pops of colour?
- Is glitter and bling a must-have for you?

CHOOSE YOUR COLOURS

Put together a colour palette – the colours you choose for your manicure can drastically change the mood of the entire look. Among your inspirational images, find colours and colour combinations that you are drawn to and imagine how they would look with your particular theme.

Light versus dark colours: Lighter colours invoke softness and tranquillity, while darker colours can look edgy, pensive and brooding.

Colour saturation: Boost your mood with vivid, bright colours. Pale, muted colours are soothing to the eye and create a peaceful look.

White: When using decal paper with clear decal film, be aware that any designs with areas of white will appear clear when placed onto the nail. You can add white later on by colouring in the decal in those areas with a thin brush and white nail polish.

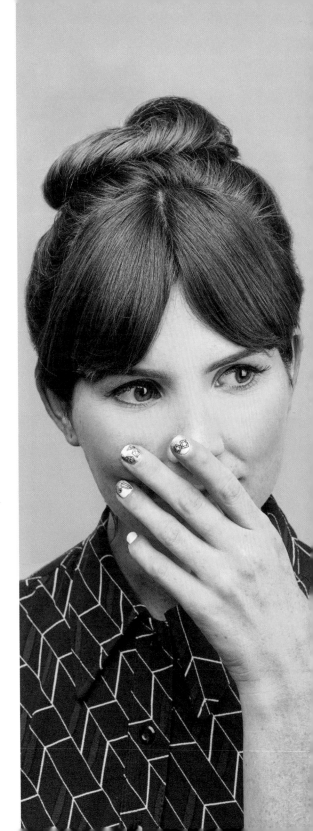

MAP OUT YOUR MANI

Create a design scheme for each finger of your manicure. (See Chapter 2 for blank nail templates and make copies if needed.) Bring together the relevant ideas and inspiration you have amassed. In each of the five fingernail templates, sketch out your overall design. Decide where the main nail decals will go first, then add to the manicure scheme from there. Place nail polish swatches next to your templates, jot down design notes alongside and see how your choices work together. Remember to try out some of the freestyling tips throughout the book to make your designs truly unique.

RESIZING YOUR DECALS

You will need to resize the decal designs throughout the book in order to make them the correct size for your nails. Take a look at your largest and longest nail beds – a wider, taller canvas means larger decals can be applied. However, if your nail beds are curved, decals that cover a lot of nail space may not lie flat. Use a smaller decal, or cut the decal into smaller pieces and put the pieces together like a jigsaw puzzle in order for them to lie flat on the nail beds. Measure the width and length of each fingernail for the best fit.

Other considerations: The decal designs will be mirrored when applied. When working with designs that are not symmetrical it is important to make sure you flip the image before printing it on decal paper.

What you will need:
• Printable inkjet or laser waterslide decal paper

• Inkjet or laser printer

• (For inkjet printing only) Clear acrylic spray or nail polish topcoat

• Ruler

• Scissors
• Nail varnish in colours of your choice
• Paper towel
• Plate
• Water
• Nail polish topcoat
• Tweezers

CUSTOMIZE YOUR LOOK

Add colour, shimmer and glitter to create nail decals with a metallic sheen – colour in the decals with a narrow brush and metallic or glitter nail polish. There are so many nail polish finishes, colours and textures to explore! Think about what types of finishes will complement your theme. Here are some of the possibilities:

Creme: Smooth nail colour.
Sheer: Nail colour with a transparent finish.
Metallic: Nail polish with metallic particles.
Shimmer: Nail polish with a coloured base and tiny reflective particles.
Holographic: Fine particles of glitter with a rainbow reflect.
Textured: Dries with a rough texture, can contain shimmer or glitter.
Foil: A metallic base with reflective particles.
Duochrome: Shimmer nail polish that changes into two (or more) colours depending on the reflection of light.
Flaky: Gel-based with opalescent glitter particles.
Gel: Transparent coloured polish with a glossy finish.
Matte: Nail polish that dries without shine.

Some designs in Chapter 3 include freestyle illustrations and tips about how to achieve the manicures in the photographs. Try one and you'll be freestyling in no time.

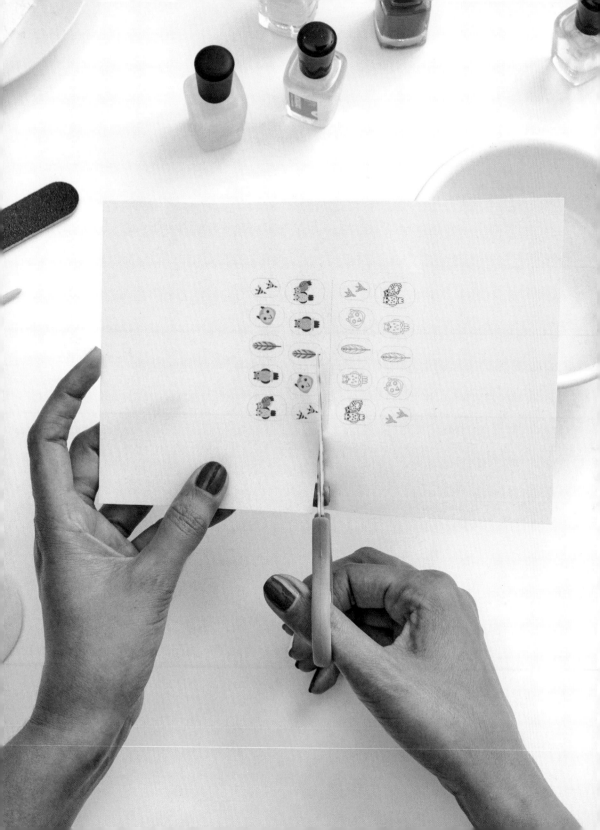

2 CREATING YOUR DECALS

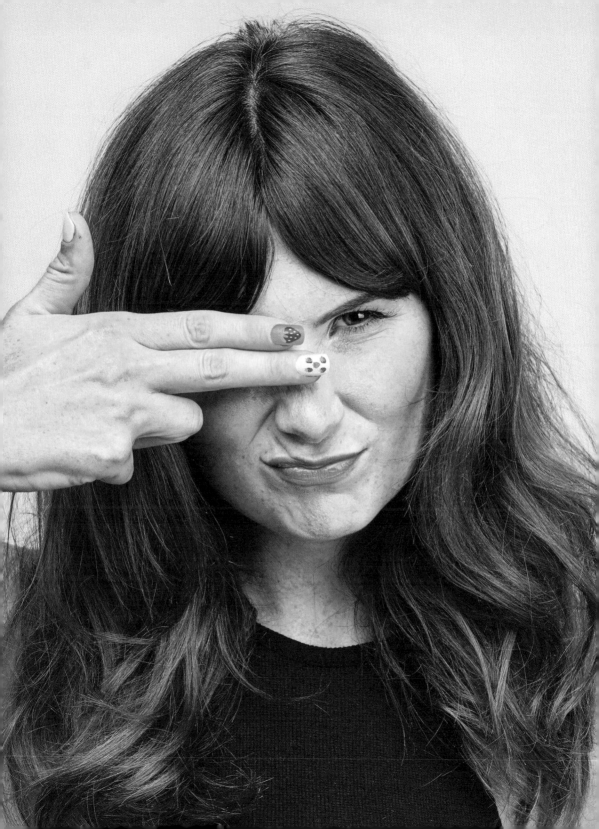

Hand-draw your decals

Hand-drawing your own nail decals from scratch can be a really fun creative experience. Remember that you do not need to draw to scale as you will be able to scan in your finished drawings and resize them to fit your nails perfectly.

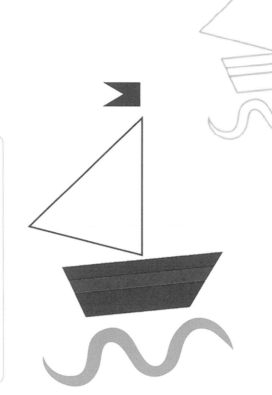

YOU WILL NEED

- Paper
- Graphite pencil
- Ruler
- Black felt-tip pen
- Pencil eraser
- Scanner
- To colour in the design: coloured pencils or markers, watercolours – or use design software to add colour

1

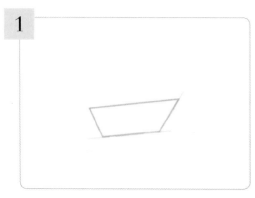

Start sketching the outline of the decal you want to create in pencil. When drawing the main elements, use a light touch.

2

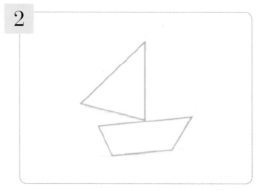

Continue to block in the proportion and angles of the design with shapes and lines to create your silhouette.

3

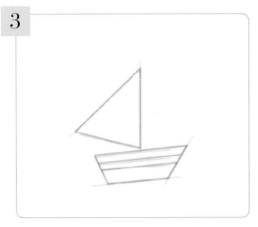

Add simple details and customization the design. Remember that very small details in your drawing may disappear when the decals are resized to fit your nail beds.

4

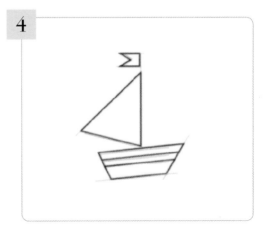

Once you end up with a design to your liking, darken the lines of the image with a black felt-tip pen. Bold, thick lines will help the decal look clear from a distance, while thinner lines will be more visible if the design is a simple one.

5

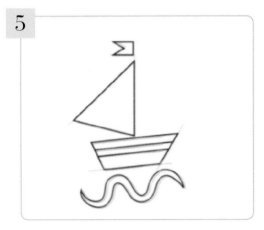

Add any background elements. When the ink is dry, remove the unnecessary pencil marks with an eraser.

6

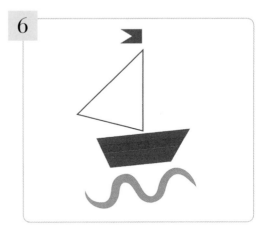

Scan the image if you plan to add colour using photo-editing software. Alternatively, colour in your design with coloured pencils, markers or paint and then scan the final coloured image.

Basic designs to draw

If you are unsure about what you want to draw, or are not confident in your drawing skills, consider these popular and simple shapes to get you started. Show your love of travel with these simple shell and flip-flop shapes. What about decorative letters using your or a loved one's initials? Or florals and feathers always make for pretty, whimsical nail designs.

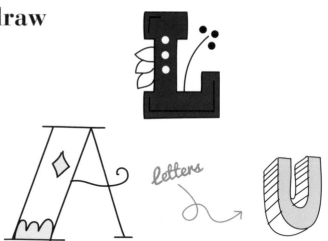

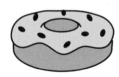

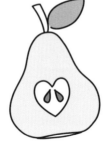

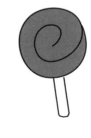

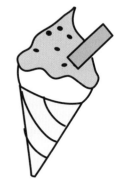

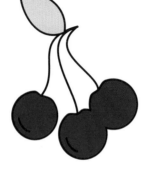

Food

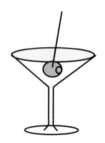

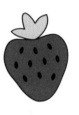

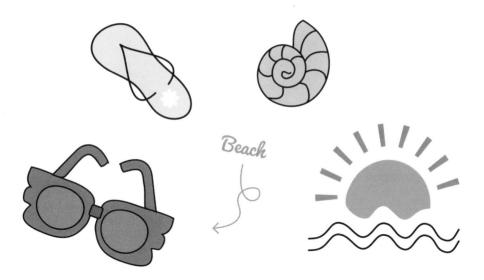

Beach

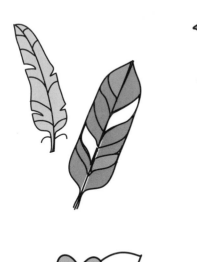

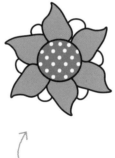

Nature

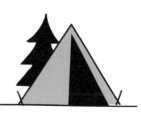

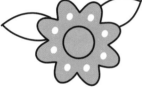

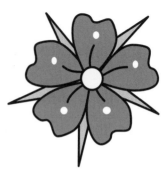

Digital designs

Take your nail decals to new, unimaginable heights of creativity using the power of computer design software. Combine images to create a miniature mosaic, or cut out portions of an image to isolate the subject. After measuring your nail beds, resizing each decal to fit your digits is child's play!

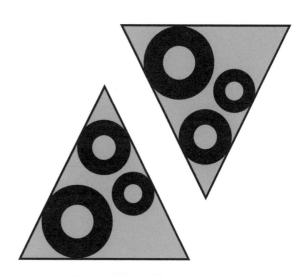

YOU WILL NEED

- Computer
- Design programme or word-processing software with image capabilities
- Photographs, scanned drawings or downloaded non-copyright images
- Ruler

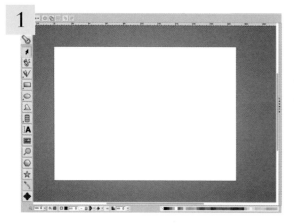

1

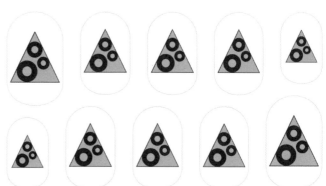

Open your design software and create a new document. The dimensions of your new document should be the same as your waterslide decal paper. If you are not using a design programme, open a word-processing programme that supports images and set the page size to match your decal paper size.

2

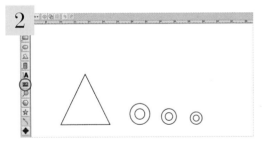

Create shapes using your software's shape tool. Use the text tool to add text or import photographs and scans using the 'insert picture' function.

3

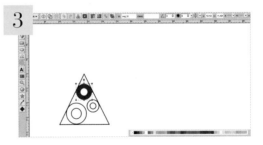

Combine elements of different images or recolour the decals for a customized look.

4

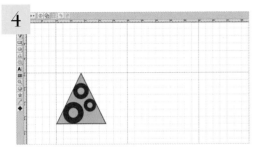

Measure your nails with a ruler. If your software allows it, use rulers and grids so you can easily determine the size of each decal.

5

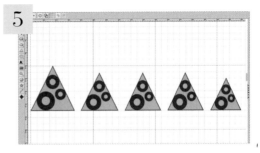

If you want repeat decals for multiple fingers, create image duplicates and resize the decals to fit the various sizes of your nails. If your nail beds are curved, cut the decal into small pieces and put it together like a jigsaw puzzle in order for the pieces to lie flat.

6

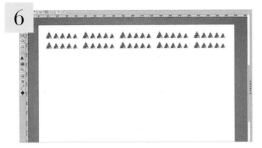

If you are unable to fill up an entire sheet of paper, arrange the images in straight rows at the top of the page. This way you can save the rest of the sheet for another time.

7

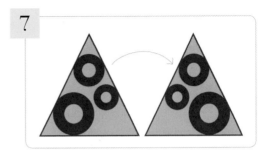

When your images are ready to print, flip them so that they mirror the original designs. This will ensure that the decals are right-side up on the nails.

Print & seal your decals

Your decal designs are complete! Now it's time to turn your ideas into reality by printing your designs onto waterslide decal paper. If your designs are not looking quite as you had hoped once you have printed them out, don't be afraid to go back and adjust colours or details as necessary to get a finished design you are happy to wear.

YOU WILL NEED

- Printable inkjet or laser waterslide decal paper
- Inkjet or laser printer
- (For inkjet printing only) Clear acrylic spray or nail polish topcoat

DECAL PAPER

Choose the type of waterslide decal paper you would like to use. There are two main types you can purchase, in craft shops or from online retailers, based on the kind of printer you have: inkjet or laser. Keep in mind that different decal papers can also have various types of decal film: some decal papers will consist of white backing paper with a clear film, others have white backing paper with an opaque white film.

If you have the option to choose clear or white film, think about your decal design colours and how much transparency you would like. If you are printing on clear-film decal paper and you have white in your decal design, that area of the decal will appear clear. Colours will be transparent, and any background colours in your nail design will show through the decal. For colours to appear bright, it's best to apply transparent film decals over white or light colours. If you are printing on white-film decal paper, the decal will be opaque and the colours will appear brighter. The downside of using white-film decal paper is that you will have to cut closely around the borders of the decal to remove excess white film around your design.

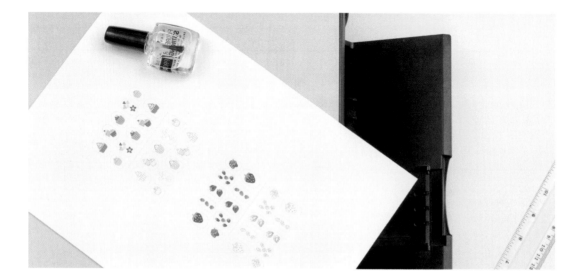

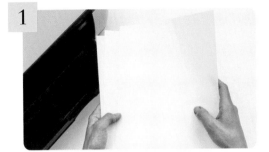

1

Determine what type of printer you will be using: inkjet or laser. If you are working with an inkjet printer, you will need to apply either a clear acrylic spray or nail polish topcoat to the printed decals before applying to your nails. Since inkjet printer ink is water soluble, a protective layer of acrylic spray or topcoat is necessary to prevent the decal ink from dissolving when the waterslide decal paper is immersed in water. Decals printed with a laser printer will not need this extra step.

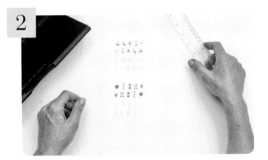

2

Before printing, measure your nail beds and adjust the decal sizes accordingly. Print out a test page on ordinary paper to see how true-to-life the colours are, and alter the decal size if the test decal does not fit. You can also adjust the brightness and/or colour saturation in your design software if needed.

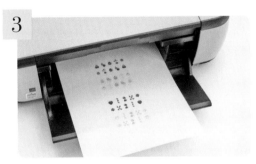

3

Once the decal sizing and colours are to your liking, place a sheet of decal paper in your printer so that your designs will print on the glossy side of your waterslide decal paper. Refer to the paper manufacturer's instructions for guidance. Verify the decal paper dimensions in your design software's 'print' function. Print out your decals and wait a few minutes for the ink to dry.

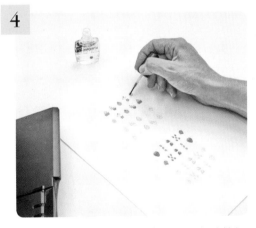

4

Remember to seal your decals if you are using inkjet decal paper (see Step 1 above). If you are printing a small number of decals, seal them with a layer of nail polish topcoat. If you are printing out a large amount, apply a clear acrylic spray coat instead. You can find this product at any craft or hardware shop, and any clear acrylic spray coat will work. Spray your printed decal sheet evenly until the sheet has a shine (approximately two to three coats). Allow one hour to dry and set before cutting.

Photocopy your decals

If you do not have a computer available for uploading and printing your decals, use a photocopier to scan the original images before printing them onto waterslide decal paper.

TIPS

- If your design includes text or can not be reversed, photocopy your design onto a plastic vellum or overhead transparency sheet. You then photocopy the reverse side of this sheet onto your decal paper, so the design will be the right side up when applied.

- Each time you photocopy your decals, the image quality will decrease. To avoid this, limit the number of copies you make.

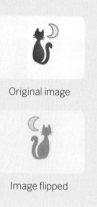

Original image

Image flipped

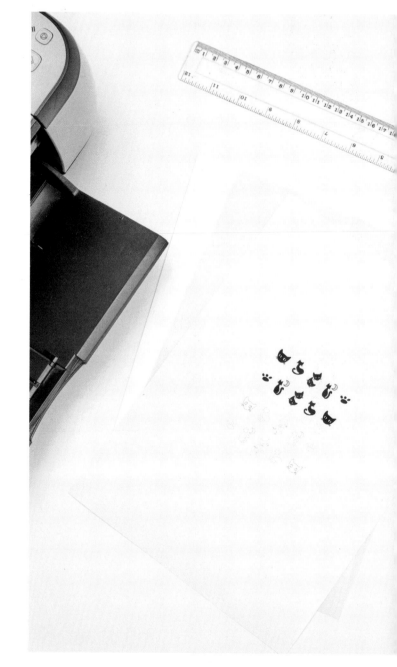

YOU WILL NEED

- Images for photocopying
- Inkjet or laser photocopier
- Ruler
- Inkjet or laser waterslide decal paper
- Plastic vellum or overhead transparency sheet

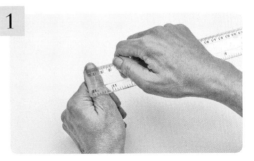

Measure your nail bed with a ruler to determine the required size of the nail decal outlines. Repeat this for different nail sizes that you wish to add to the page.

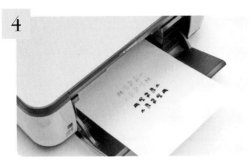

Use the photocopier's enlarge or reduce functions to resize the decals to fit your nail beds.

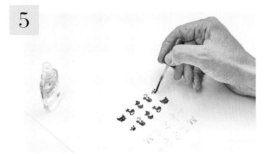

Photocopy a test page onto plain paper to verify the decal sizing.

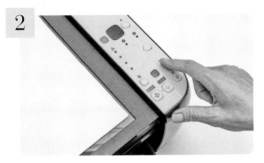

Once the decal sizes are correct, photocopy your designs onto waterslide decal paper on the correct side and let the ink dry completely.

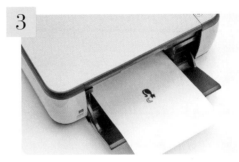

If your photocopier prints with ink, you will need to seal your decals. See 'Print & seal your decals' on pages 22–3 for instructions.

Apply your decals

Once you have chosen and prepared your decal designs, it's time to apply them to your nails. This process is very quick and easy, so your custom mani will be ready in a flash!

YOU WILL NEED

- Nail base coat
- Nail polish
- Scissors
- Waterslide decals
- Paper towel
- Plate
- Water
- Nail polish topcoat
- Tweezers

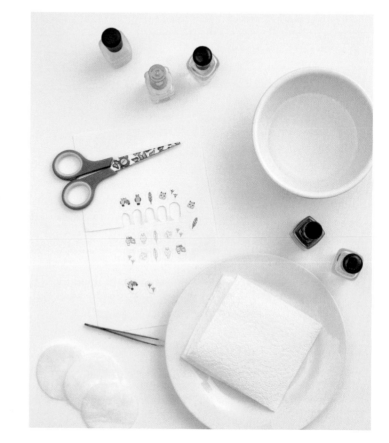

1

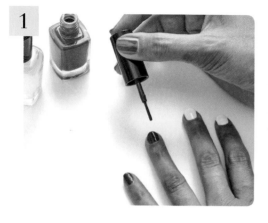

Apply a base coat to protect your natural nails and to help the nail polish adhere. Once the base coat is dry, apply two coats of nail polish, letting each layer dry completely before applying the next. (If you are using glitter nail polish, the bumpy surface may not allow the decals to lie flat. In this instance, apply a layer of topcoat over the glitter nail polish to help smooth out the surface.)

2

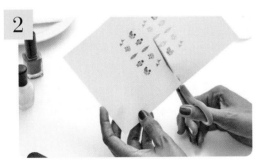

Once you have printed your decals, check that the images are reversed. (When applied to the nails, they will have the correct orientation.) Cut out your decals, trimming as closely to the image outlines as you can.

3

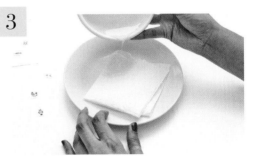

Place a paper towel onto a plate. Wet the paper towel with water.

4

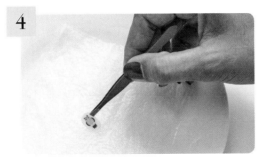

Place your decal onto the wet paper towel, with the paper backing facing down.

5

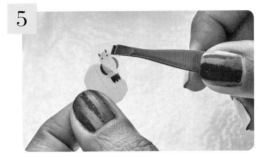

Once the paper backing has soaked through, slide the paper away from the decal and pat it dry.

6

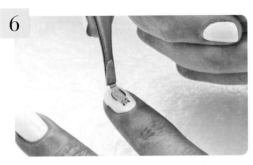

Very carefully apply the decal to your nail with the tweezers.

7

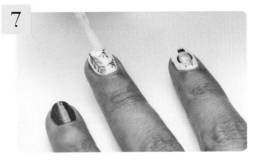

To set the decal in place, apply a single layer of clear topcoat over the nail and the decal.

Decal templates

Draw your own designs into these templates, then scan them in or photocopy them onto your decal paper. Remember to resize them (as per the photocopier instructions on pages 24-25) so they fit your nail beds perfectly.

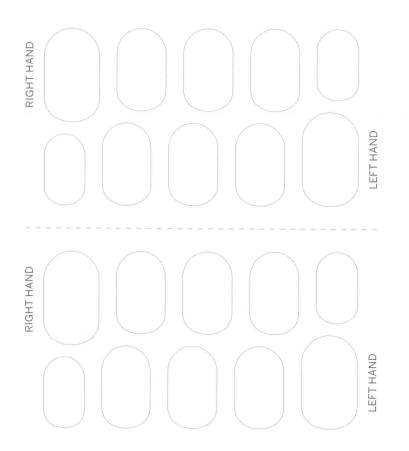

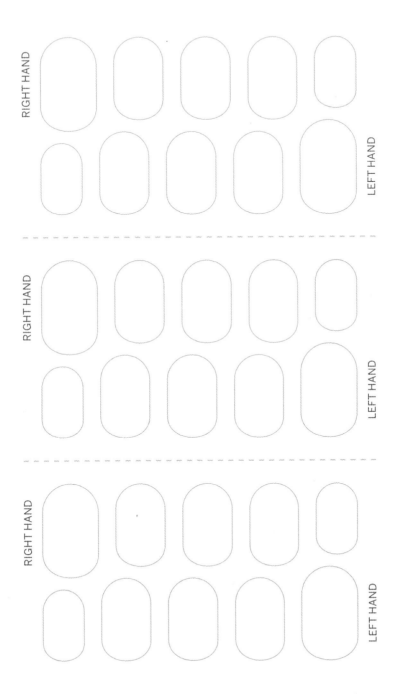

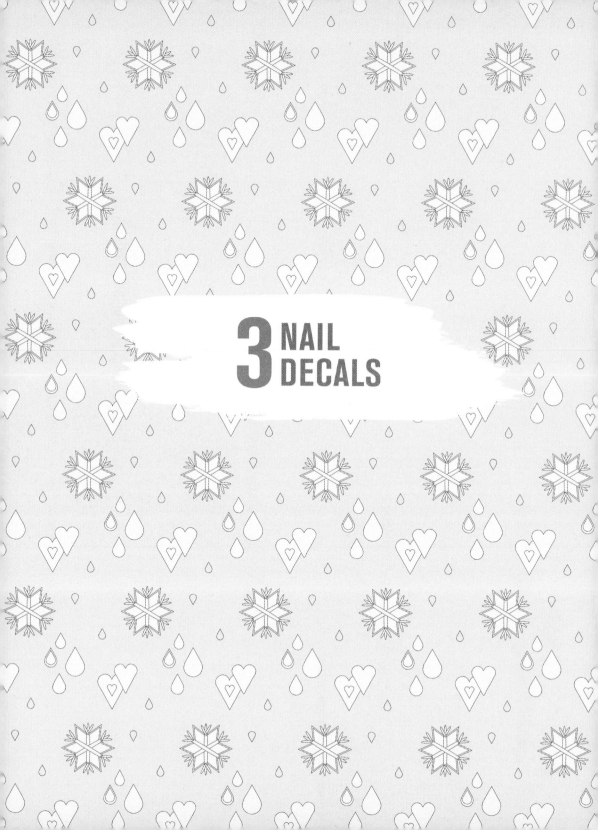

3 NAIL DECALS

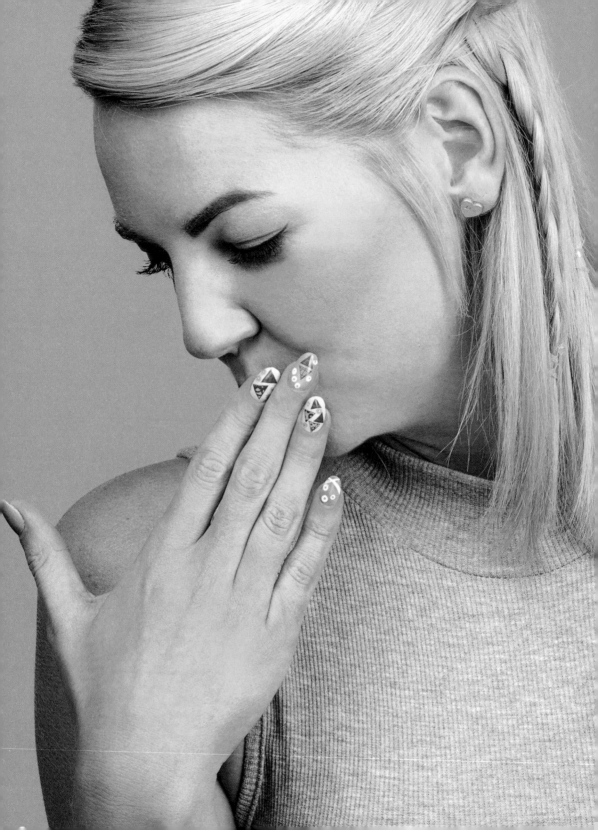

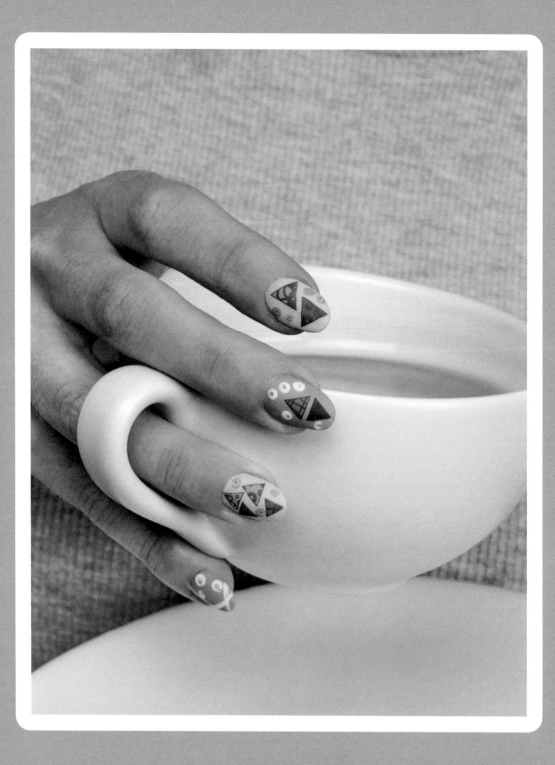

Patterned Triangles

A striking geometric print in soft, muted colours looks fresh and modern, and can lend itself well to any occasion. A blend of classic and graphic, this design keeps the mood bright when paired with crisp white nail polish. Or wear with opaque nudes and pastels for a coordinated look that will make those shapes pop.

TIPS

- If you have chosen to colour in your nail decals, use all opaque nail colours to make the shapes pop.

- Bold graphics pair beautifully with metallics. Paint one or two nails in a complementary metallic nail polish to add visual balance to your mani.

FREESTYLE TIPS

- Add contrasting shapes to the backgrounds to really make these geometrics pop. Polka dots can be painted freehand using a hair grip dipped in your nail polish colour of choice.

- Try creating accent nails with curved lines at the tips. The lines can be applied using a thin synthetic brush – and a very steady hand!

TO SCAN (THEN RESIZE)

TO COLOUR (THEN RESIZE)

TO FREESTYLE

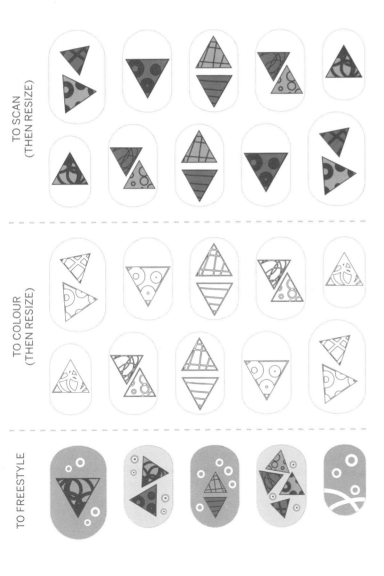

TO DOWNLOAD

tinyurl.com/ hzpo5ao

Graphic Florals

Florals do not have to be obviously girly. Make them more edgy with graphic shapes that sharpen the look. Not just for spring or summer days, these striking florals will last well into autumn and winter – just update the colour combos to match the season. Pair with accents of metallics for added impact.

POTENTIAL COLOURWAYS

- White, silver, fuchsia pink
- Pink, purple, orange, teal
- Gold, red, green
- Silver, pale blue, white

TO SCAN
(THEN RESIZE)

TO COLOUR
(THEN RESIZE)

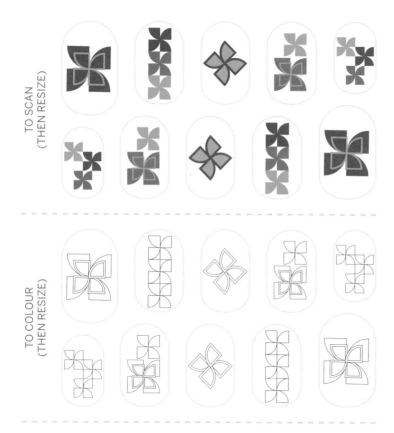

TO DOWNLOAD

tinyurl.com/
hzpo5ao

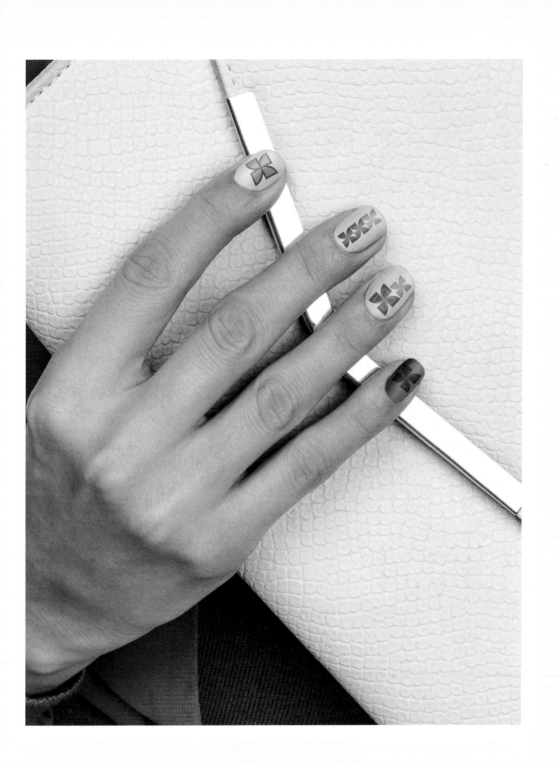

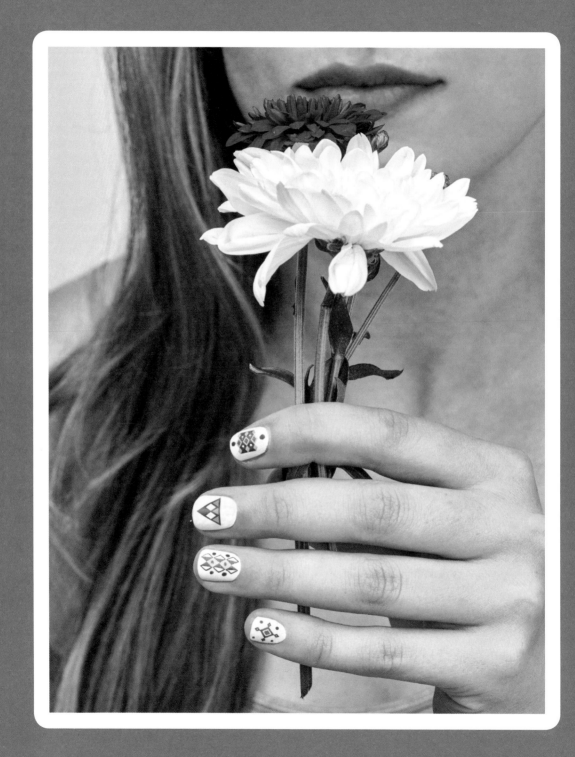

Traditional

Add impact to your nails with bold tribal tattoos! These high-contrast designs can include intricate geometric patterns or take inspiration from their original Polynesian roots. Paint background nails white for a fresh look to breeze through summer.

TIPS

• Layer simple black decals over ombré (shaded) nails for a stunning effect.

Add a tribal French tip:

1. Square off the nail tips with a nail file.

2. Cut off a linear section of tribal print.

3. Apply decal to the nail tip.

TO SCAN (THEN RESIZE)

TO COLOUR (THEN RESIZE)

TO DOWNLOAD

tinyurl.com/hzpo5ao

Boho

Trendy tribal-print nails are ideal for boho summer festivals! In bright neon hues and contrasting dark line work, these distinctive prints work wonderfully with gold metallic accents. These designs are perfect for soaking up your favourite music vibes in a field, or for some serious poolside lounging.

POTENTIAL COLOURWAYS

- White, gold, orange, pink, yellow
- Purple, gold, black
- Silver, blue, white
- Teal, pink, gold

TO SCAN (THEN RESIZE)

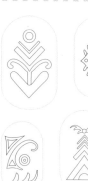
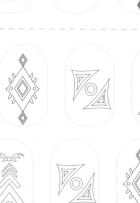

TO COLOUR (THEN RESIZE)

TO DOWNLOAD

tinyurl.com/ hzpo5ao

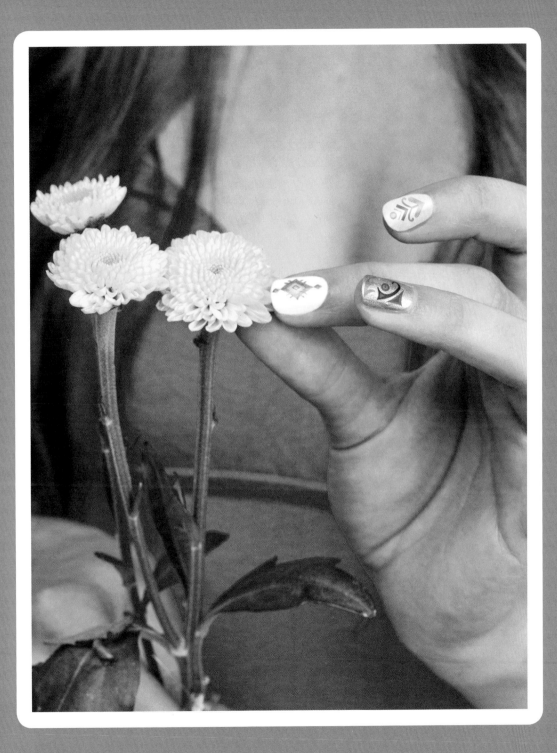

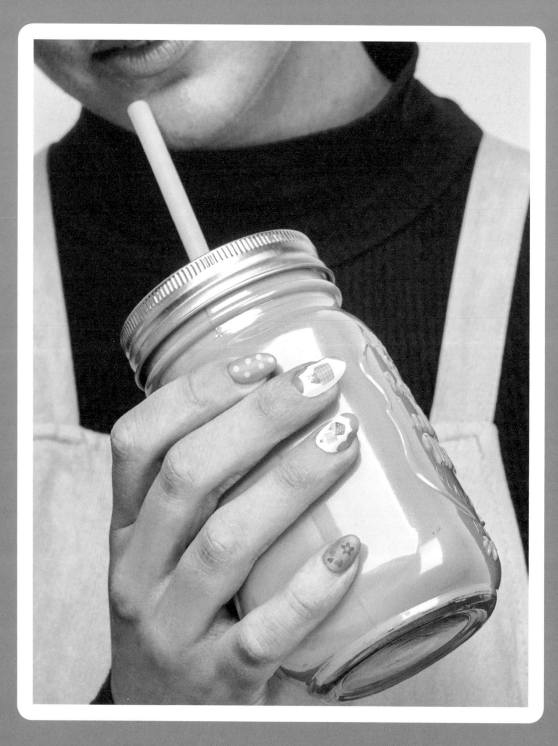

Cupcakes

Need a pick-me-up? A sweet treat wouldn't hurt! Adorable desserts such as cupcakes, macarons and doughnuts are always on trend when it comes to nail art. Why not try mixing in some patterns to make your nails even more unique? These hearts and flowers in pastel shades bring added cute factor!

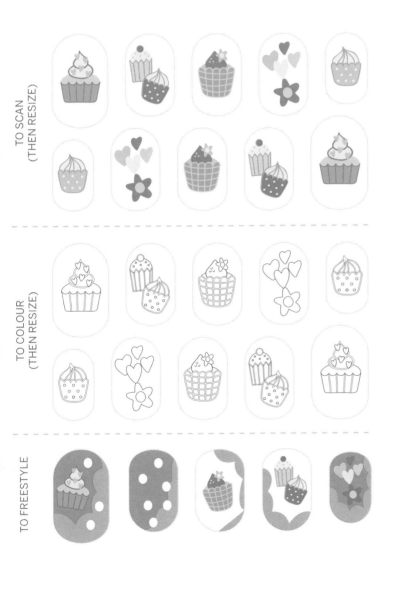

TO SCAN
(THEN RESIZE)

TO COLOUR
(THEN RESIZE)

TO FREESTYLE

TIPS

- Paint each nail in a soft rainbow of pastel colours. Add cupcake decals on each nail in colours that contrast with the background polish.

Feminine polka dots work well with sweets:

1. Apply a pastel base colour to the nail first.
2. Take a hair grip and add some white nail polish to its round end.
3. Dab the end of the hair grip onto the nail to create polka dots.

FREESTYLE TIPS

- Some freehand painting enhances these cute cupcakes beautifully. Try using a thin synthetic brush to create a scalloped frame around your nails for a truly feminine finish.

TO DOWNLOAD

tinyurl.com/
hzpo5ao

41

Pizza Slices

We all have our vices – celebrate your love for all things yummy with kitschy food designs. Fast-food prints are a fun 90s throwback; pair cheesy pizza slices with a black-and-white colourway for a grungy skater feel, or paint background nails in neutrals to make these delicious designs look good enough to eat!

POTENTIAL COLOURWAYS

- Red, yellow, orange, black, nude
- Green, red, gold
- Red, orange, green, white
- Purple, orange, green, red

TO SCAN
(THEN RESIZE)

TO COLOUR
(THEN RESIZE)

TO DOWNLOAD

tinyurl.com/
hzpo5ao

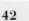

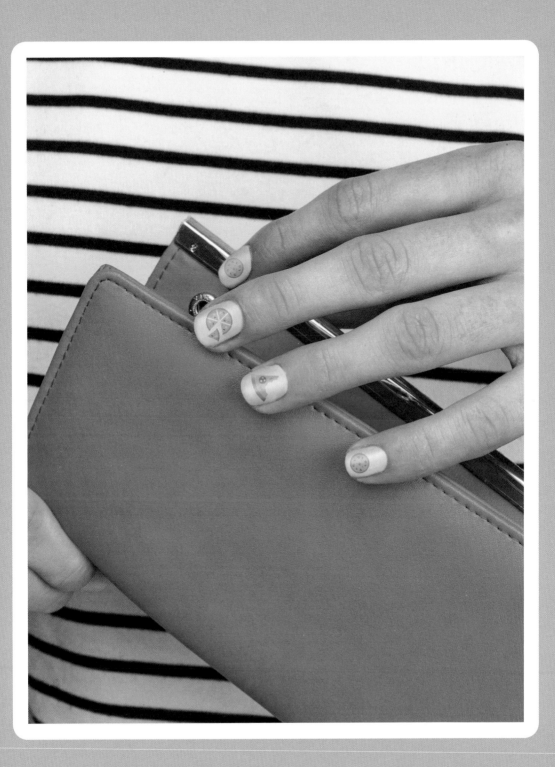

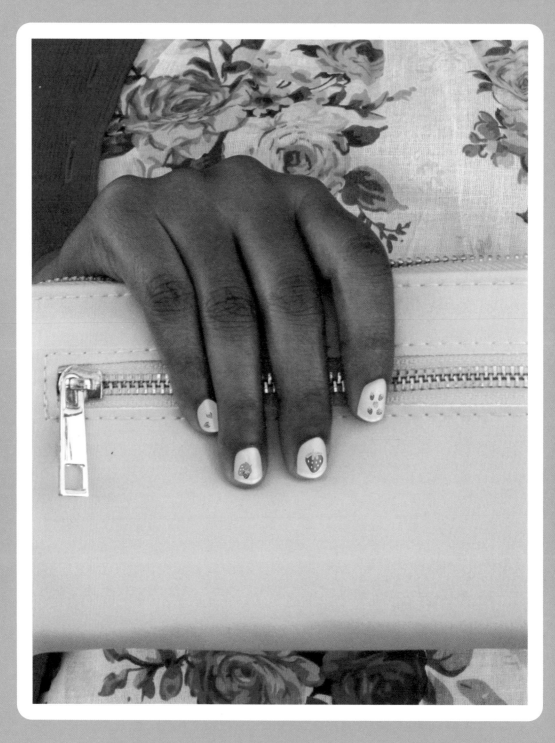

Strawberries

Feeling sweet? This petite fruit exudes playful feminine appeal. Paint your nails bright yellow for a zingy background, perfect for long summer days, or try a soft muted tone for a classic manicure with a twist. Strawberry fields forever!

TO SCAN (THEN RESIZE)

TO COLOUR (THEN RESIZE)

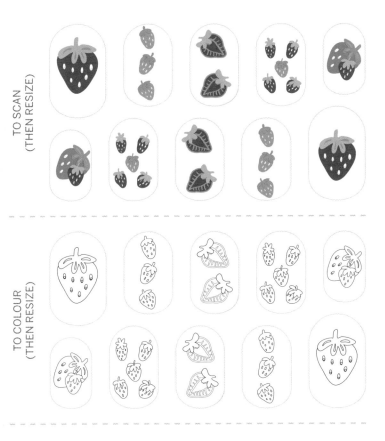

TO DOWNLOAD

tinyurl.com/ hzpo5ao

Watermelon

Just add watermelon! Fruit-inspired nails are the perfect juicy addition to summer fashion trends. Festive watermelon slices pack a punch and are reminiscent of summer picnics and lazy days by the pool. Pair with bright accent nails for a mouthwatering mani!

POTENTIAL COLOURWAYS

- Red, orange, sky blue
- Spring green, baby pink, white
- Nude, pink, green, black
- Fuchsia pink, green, yellow, white

FREESTYLE TIPS

- Add interest to accent nails by painting the watermelon skin close to the tip using a thin synthetic brush, as shown on the little finger.
- You could playfully mimic watermelon seeds by painting a scattering of tiny dark dots on half of another nail, using the tip of a very thin brush or a toothpick.

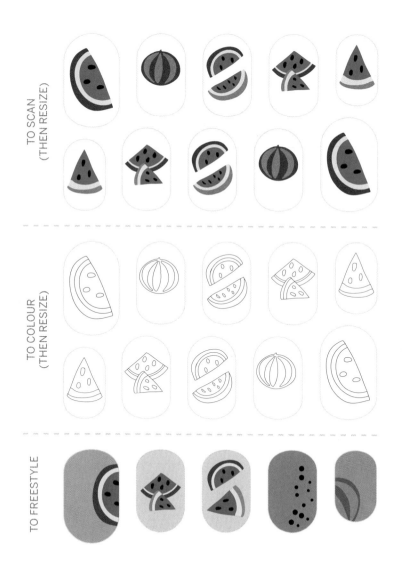

TO SCAN
(THEN RESIZE)

TO COLOUR
(THEN RESIZE)

TO FREESTYLE

TO DOWNLOAD

tinyurl.com/
hzpo5ao

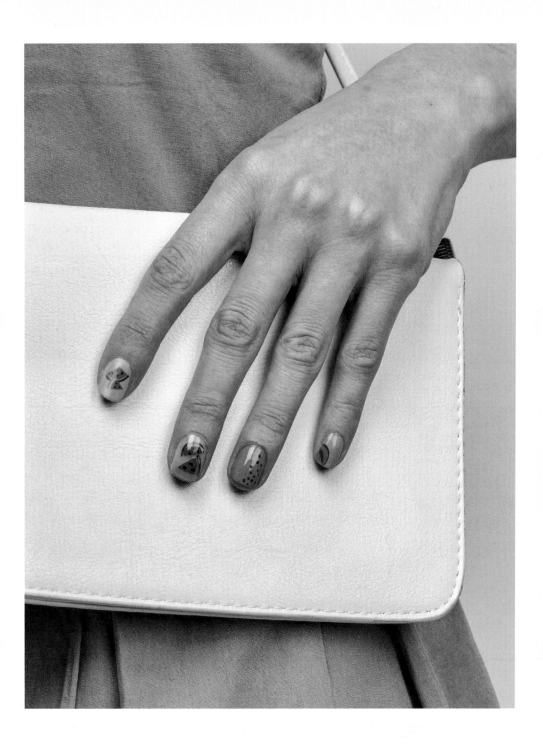

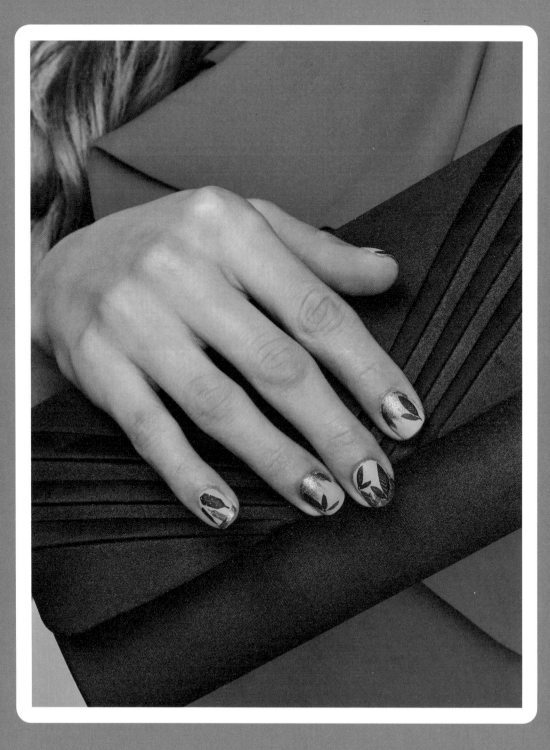

Monochrome

In a monochrome colourway, you can leave the feathers as they are for a simple, sophisticated look, or colour in the feathers with a nail polish of your choice. Add accents of silver metallic polish for an instant injection of sharp glamour.

TIPS

- Try monochrome decals and a bright background for a hint of fun behind the glamour, or colour in your own decals in peacock shades of green and blue.

Can't decide on a single shade? Make ombré French tips:

- Gather five nail polishes in a single shade from light to dark – for example, light blue to dark blue.
- From thumb to little finger, apply a thin French tip using each colour in order, from light to dark.

FREESTYLE TIPS

- Metallic silver is perfect for a monochrome colourway. Create a colour-gradient background by dabbing silver metallic polish onto the bottom edge of your nail with a make-up sponge.
- Add French tips in silver for a sharp, sophisticated finish.

TO SCAN (THEN RESIZE)

TO COLOUR (THEN RESIZE)

TO FREESTYLE

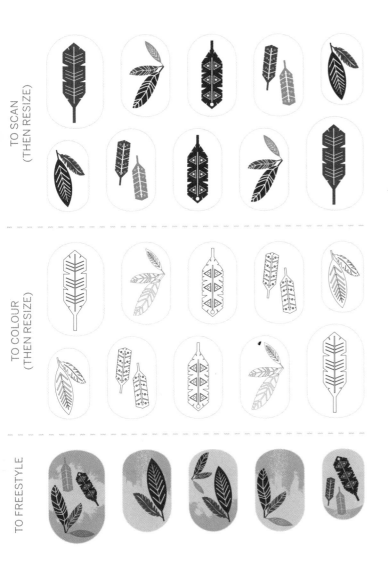

TO DOWNLOAD

tinyurl.com/ hzpo5ao

Colourful

Feathers are not just for costumes or haute couture. Whimsical and breezy, feather motifs are beautiful when paired with nail art in summer and autumn colour palettes. Why not try mixing in patterns such as delicate gold polka dots to enhance this elegant mani?

POTENTIAL COLOURWAYS

• Purple, sky blue
• Blue, pink, purple
• Dark blue, white, grey
• Blue, emerald green, teal
• Nude, pink, purple
• Pale blue, dark blue, silver

TO SCAN (THEN RESIZE)

TO COLOUR (THEN RESIZE)

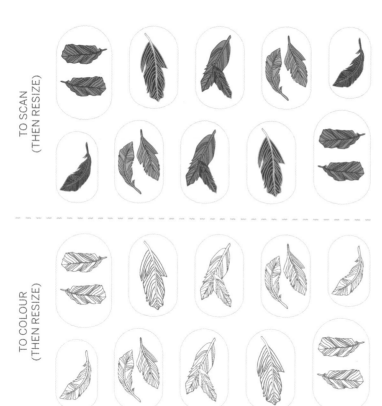

TO DOWNLOAD

tinyurl.com/hzpo5ao

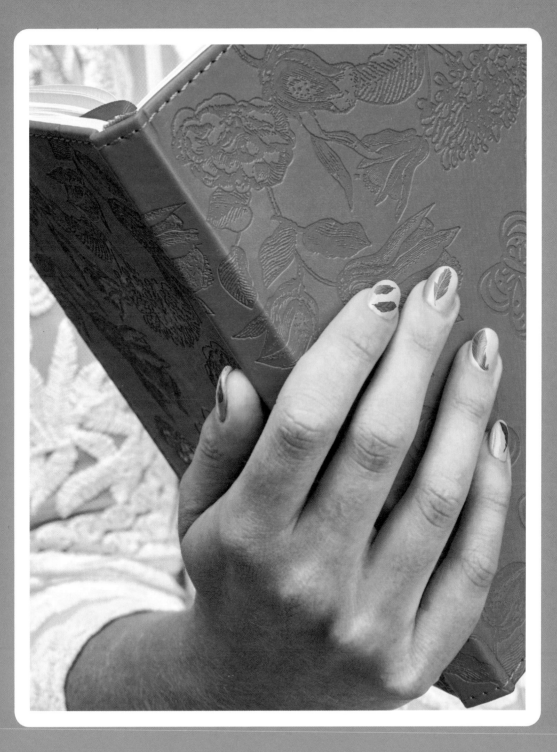

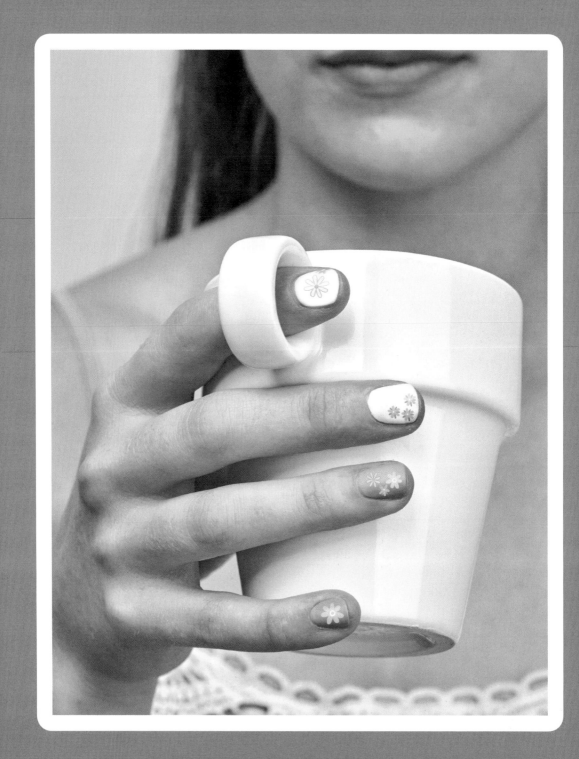

Daisy

Sunny daisy motifs are quaint and pretty yet also reminiscent of 90s fashion. This playful print is feminine enough without being too serious. Pair daisies with sky-blue nail polish and contrasting black-and-white stripes for florals that pack a punch, or wear with pastels and white for a soft, fresh look.

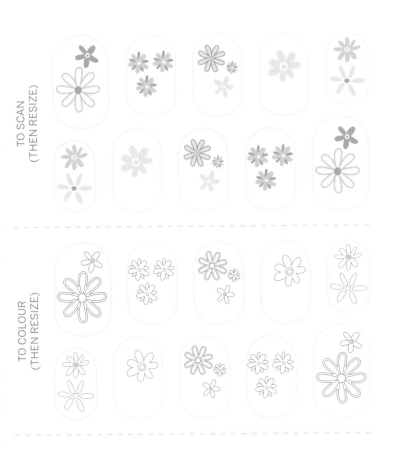

TIPS

- By switching your colour palette to autumn hues or festive berry shades, floral designs can bloom throughout the changing seasons.

To create simple vines and leaves:

1. Use a narrow synthetic brush dipped in green nail polish to create greenery.

2. Rest your painting hand on your working surface and apply the brush to the nail in norrow, curved strokes to make the vines.

3. Apply short diagonal strokes along the vines to make the leaves.

TO DOWNLOAD

tinyurl.com/ hzpo5ao

Botanical

Florals are a tried and tested nail art staple, perfect for both everyday wear and special occasions. Feature your favourite blooms with meandering stems and leaves to flex your flower power. Add DIY floral shapes alongside your decals to make your mani truly unique.

POTENTIAL COLOURWAYS

- Pink, grey, white, silver, gold
- Pale green, dark green, pink, red
- Gold, emerald green, Fuchsia pink
- Green, purple, pink, silver

TO SCAN (THEN RESIZE)

TO COLOUR (THEN RESIZE)

TO DOWNLOAD

tinyurl.com/
hzpo5ao

54

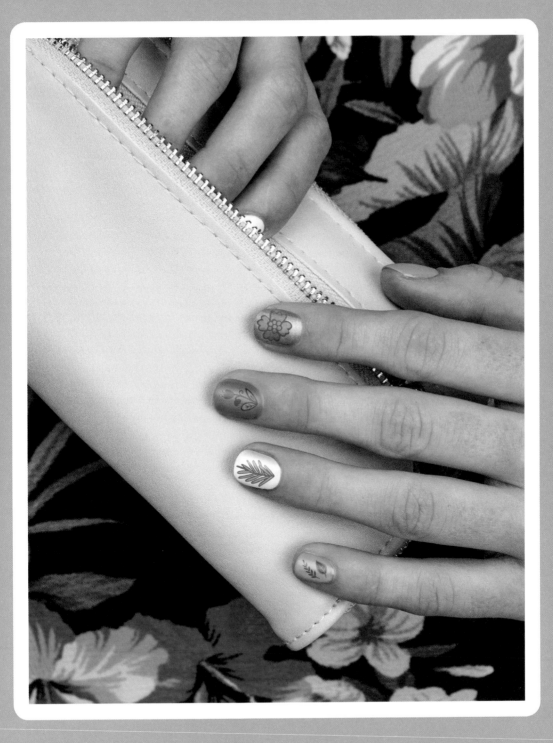

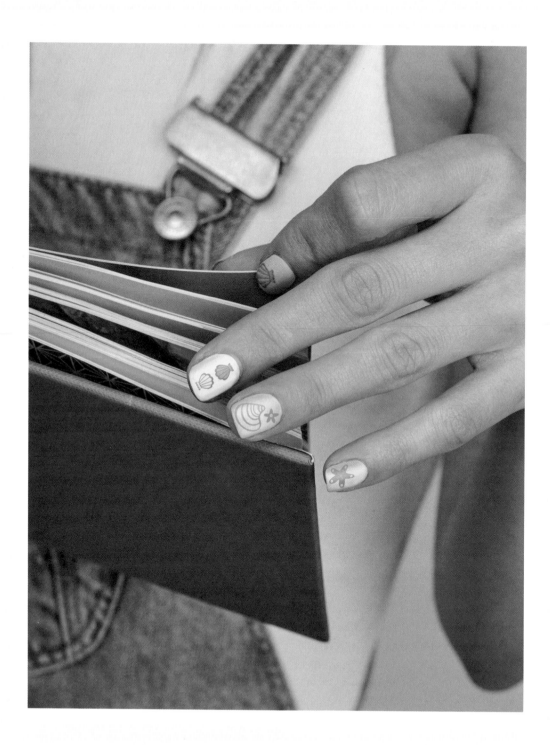

Seashells and Starfish

Seashell and starfish nail art seems to make a comeback every summer, with no sign of going out of style. Pair marine life with shades of blue, white and sea-foam green to make waves with your nail art. Perfect for lazy summer days on the beach!

TIPS

To paint nautical stripes:

1. Dip a long, narrow, synthetic brush into navy blue nail polish.

2. Wipe off any excess nail polish from the brush to prevent drips.

3. Rest your wrist on a table while holding the brush.

4. To create a steady line, apply the brush to the nail surface and hold it still while slowly rotating the nail you are painting.

TO SCAN (THEN RESIZE)

TO COLOUR (THEN RESIZE)

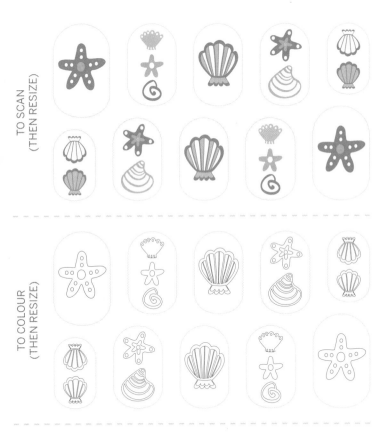

TO DOWNLOAD

tinyurl.com/ hzpo5ao

Nautical

Hello, sailor! Summer months call for nautical-inspired nails. Sail away on the high seas with boats and anchors on red, blue and white nails. Add dainty metal studs or rhinestones to catch the sunlight, and finish the look with accent nails painted in nautical stripes.

TO SCAN (THEN RESIZE)

TO COLOUR (THEN RESIZE)

TO DOWNLOAD

tinyurl.com/ hzpo5ao

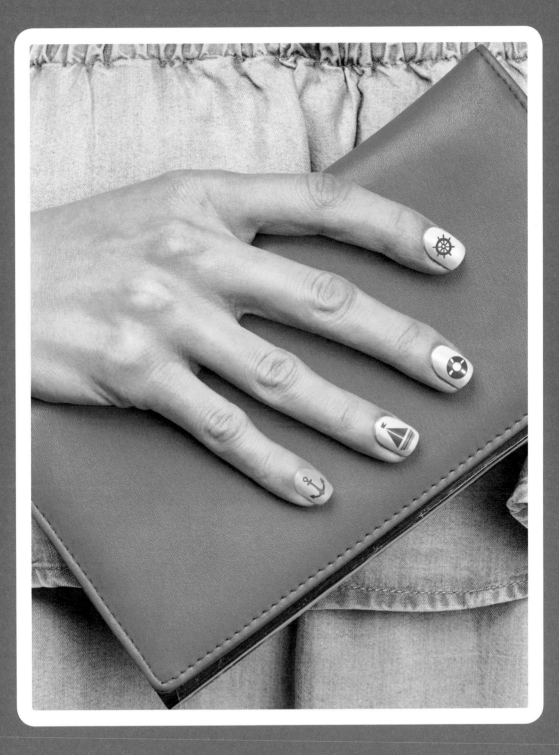

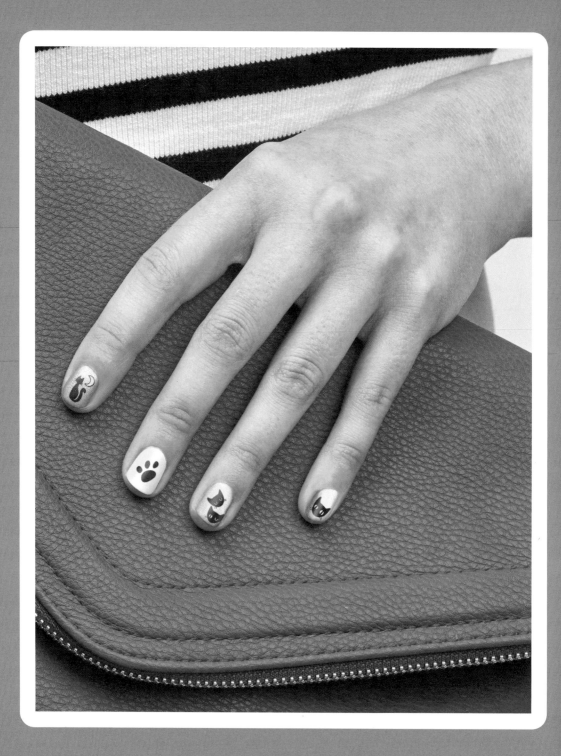

Cats

Cat-themed designs are full of playful panache and these decals are irresistibly cute. For a manicure that is absolute purrfection, enhance feline figures with paw prints and make your cat even more mysterious by adding a crescent moon in the background.

TO SCAN
(THEN RESIZE)

TO COLOUR
(THEN RESIZE)

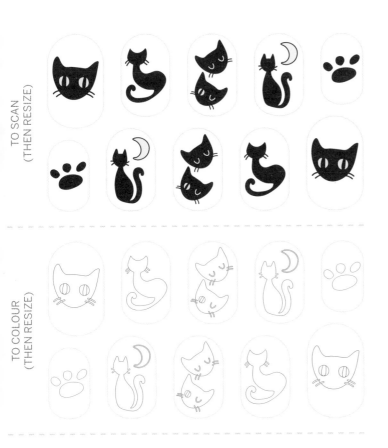

TIPS

To make a simple paw print:

1. Paint a circle about two-thirds of the way down the nail bed to make the centre of the cat's paw.

2. Dip a hair grip in black nail polish.

3. Use the hair grip and nail polish to create three smaller dots around the paw's centre to make toe prints.

To add rhinestones to the cat's eyes:

1. Dip a toothpick in some nail glue and apply it to the eyes.

2. Before the glue dries, apply a small rhinestone to each eye with tweezers.

TO DOWNLOAD

tinyurl.com/
hzpo5ao

Dogs

Express your love for your canine companion with unique and fun dog-centric decals. Quirky and charming, dog motifs are prevalent in preppy fashion trends, especially French bulldogs and dachshund silhouettes. Include paw prints for added pup appeal!

POTENTIAL COLOURWAYS

- Lavender, blue, pink, white, gold, black
- Black, white, grey, red, gold
- Gold, black, white
- Red, grey, black, white

FREESTYLE TIPS

- Paint your nails in white and finish with a delicate French tip in black to enhance the doggy details in your decals.

TO SCAN (THEN RESIZE)

TO COLOUR (THEN RESIZE)

TO FREESTYLE

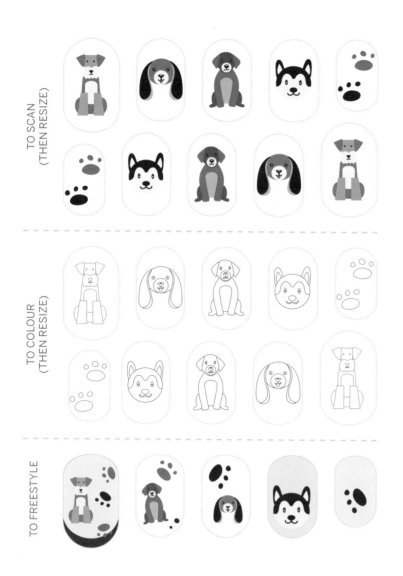

TO DOWNLOAD

tinyurl.com/ hzpo5ao

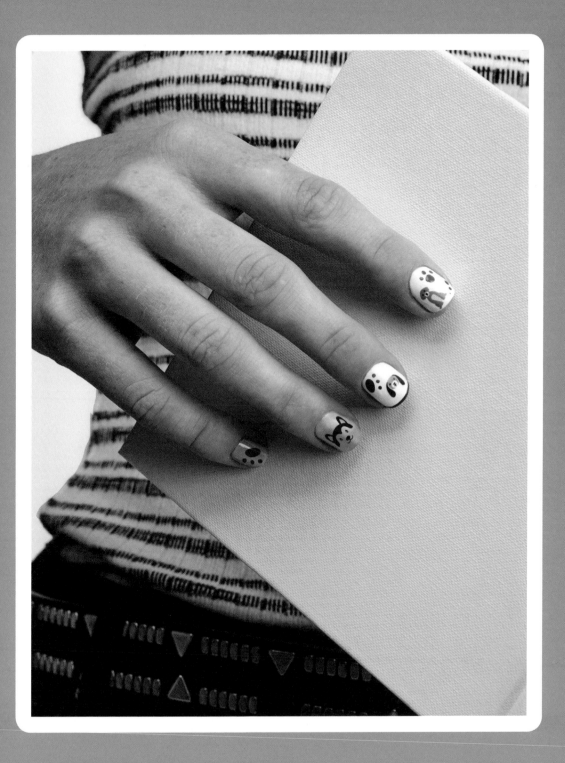

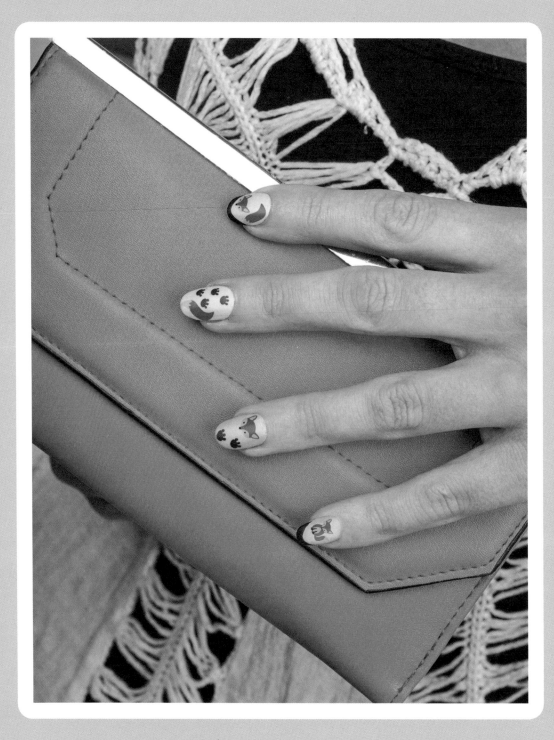

Foxes

Fairytale images of woodland foxes are perfect for autumn. Pair the fantastic fox with shades of moss green and rich berry reds and pinks, or keep the background neutral and let your foxy friends take centre stage. Bushy tails and paw prints bring added fun factor.

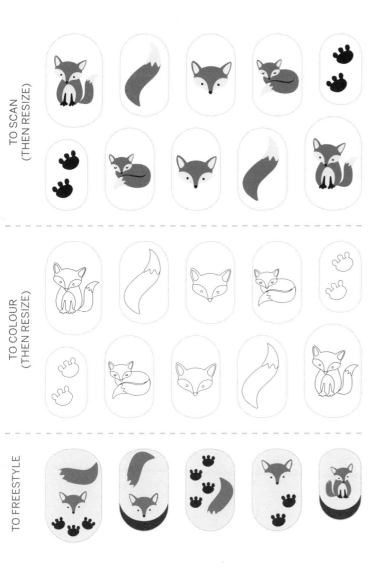

TO SCAN
(THEN RESIZE)

TO COLOUR
(THEN RESIZE)

TO FREESTYLE

TIPS

To make silhouette treescapes:

1. Paint your nail in sky blue.

2. Paint a small vertical line with black nail polish on one side of your nail.

3. Add diagonal strokes to both sides of the vertical line to create a simple tree. Add another tree next to the first.

4. To make the forest floor, apply black nail polish to the nail below your trees.

FREESTYLE TIPS

• Add dark French tips to contrast with neutral background colours and to pick out detailing in the foxy decals.

TO DOWNLOAD

tinyurl.com/
hzpo5ao

Owls

Take inspiration from creatures of the forest. The owl is a symbol of wisdom and knowledge and was a very popular home decor theme in the 70s. Today they make a quirky addition to any mani. Pair with whimsical feather motifs and metallic French tips for a modern take on a wise old friend.

POTENTIAL COLOURWAYS

- Teal, green, yellow, gold
- Turquoise, pink, purple
- Fuchsia pink, emerald green, pale green, gold
- Yellow, purple, blue, gold

FREESTYLE TIPS

- Be a night owl and take your look from daytime to evening with the addition of silver glitter French tips. These look striking against dark background hues and blend beautifully with neutrals.

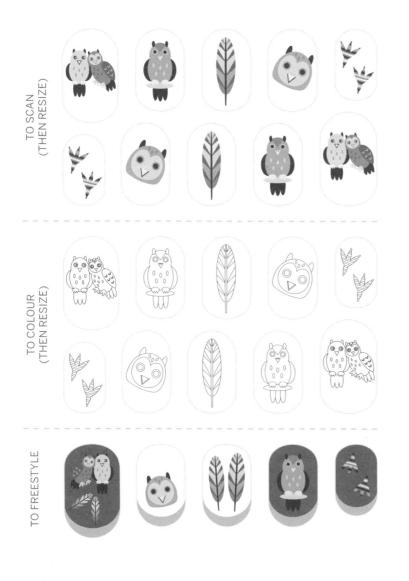

TO SCAN (THEN RESIZE)

TO COLOUR (THEN RESIZE)

TO FREESTYLE

TO DOWNLOAD

tinyurl.com/ hzpo5ao

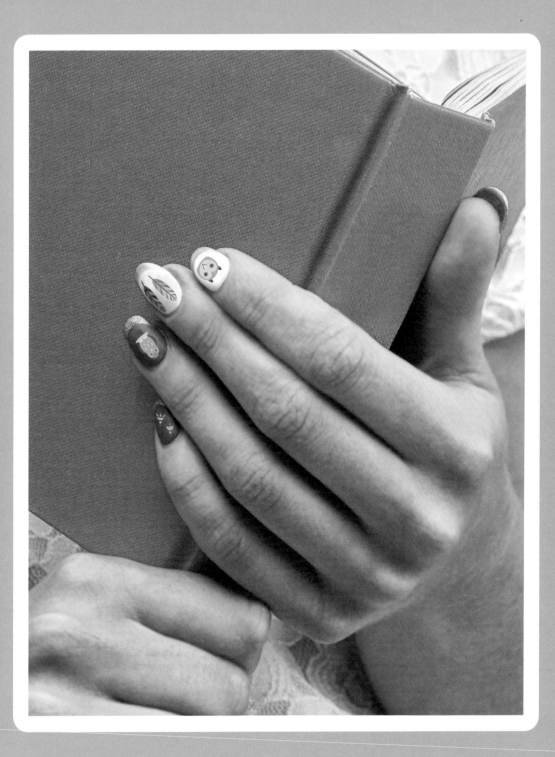

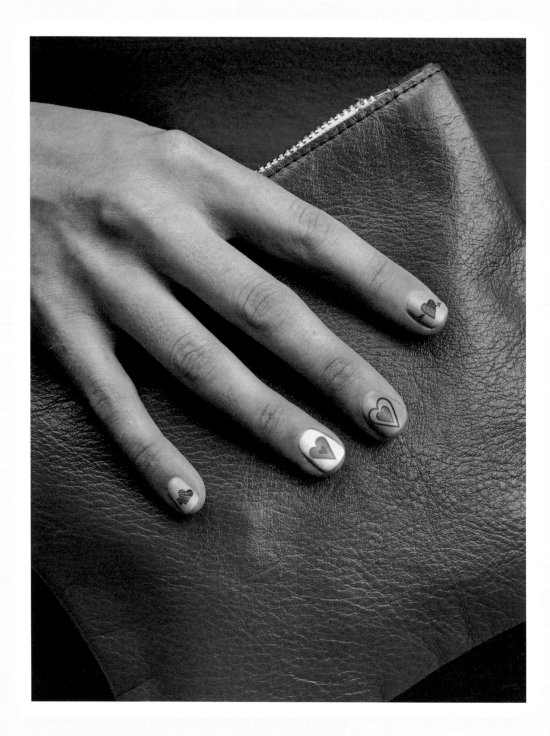

Hearts

Wear your heart on you nails with these lovely romantic decals. Sweet and playful without being overly flashy, they will work well over white, light pink or neutral shades. Design your own heart shapes alongside these decals to make this mani your own.

TIPS

To create simple heart shapes with nail polish:

1. Dip the round end of a hair grip in red nail polish.

2. Paint two dots adjacent to one another. This will be the top of the heart.

3. Dip a toothpick in the same red nail polish and draw a 'V' underneath the two dots to complete the heart.

TO SCAN (THEN RESIZE)

TO COLOUR (THEN RESIZE)

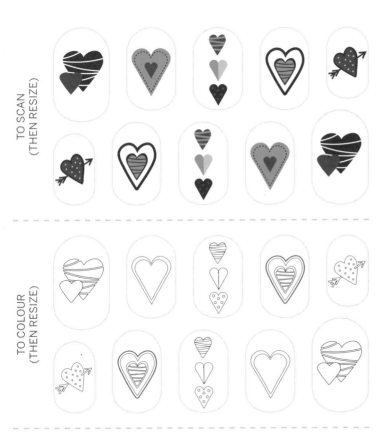

TO DOWNLOAD

tinyurl.com/hzpo5ao

Lips

Cast a love spell with these red lipstick kisses. A red lip is a classic beauty trend that will never go out of style. Cover your nails with lip prints in various sizes and finish them off with accents of glitter nail polish for added sparkle. It's time to kiss boring nail art goodbye!

POTENTIAL COLOURWAYS

- Red, pink, white
- Fuchsia pink, pale pink, pink glitter
- Red, white
- Red, orange, nude

FREESTYLE TIPS

- Add a little glam to your nails by using pink glitter polish on your little finger.
- Use the pink glitter polish to add a French tip to one of your other nails to tie the look together.

TO SCAN (THEN RESIZE)

TO COLOUR (THEN RESIZE)

TO FREESTYLE

TO DOWNLOAD

tinyurl.com/ hzpo5ao

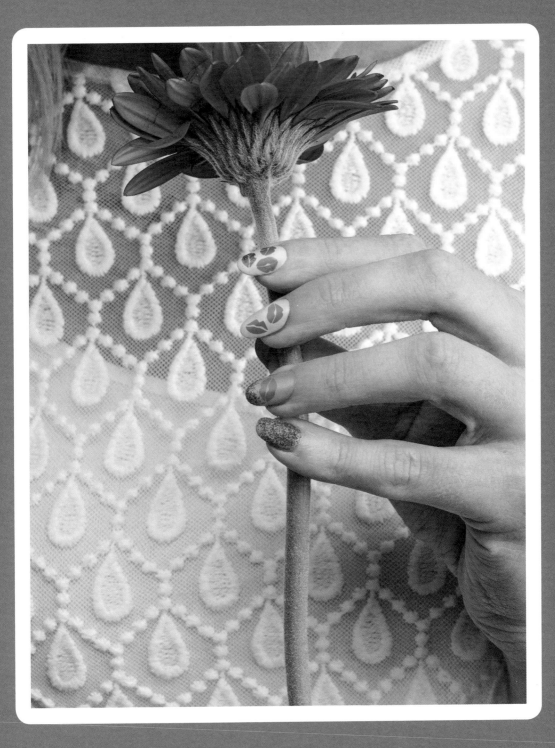

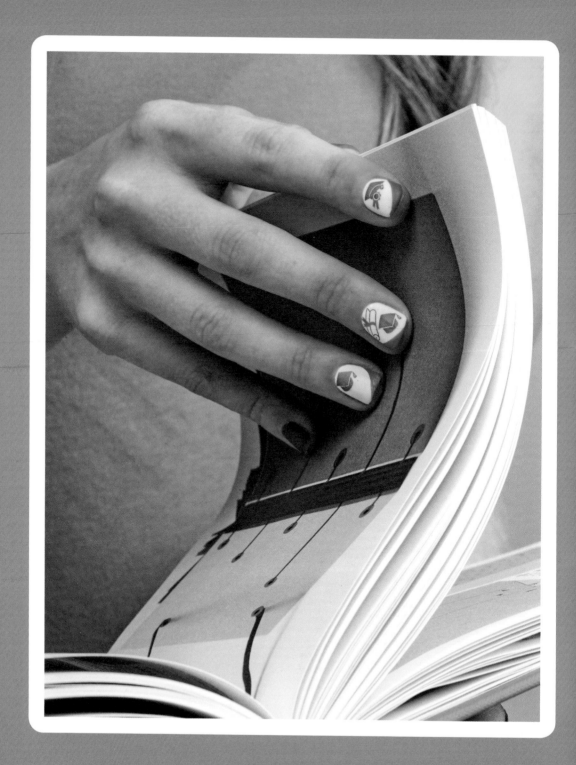

Graduation

Graduate your style with college-inspired designs and celebrate your academic milestones with diplomas and mortarboards for a scholarly look that sends you straight to the head of the class! For added flair, why not finish the design with coloured French tips painted at an angle?

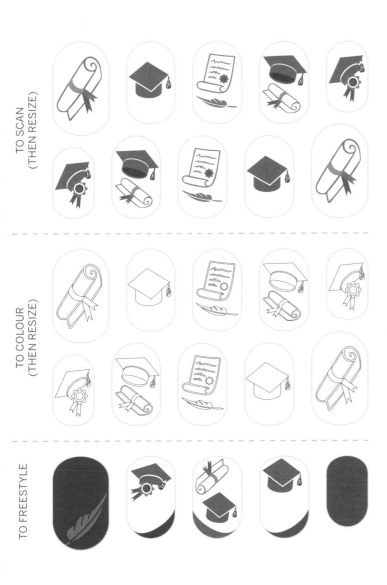

TO SCAN
(THEN RESIZE)

TO COLOUR
(THEN RESIZE)

TO FREESTYLE

TIPS

Create a notebook-paper background for your scholarly nail decals:

1. Paint your nail white.

2. Dip a narrow brush in a light blue nail polish, and add horizontal stripes to the nail.

3. Clean off the brush and dip it in a red nail polish. Paint one vertical line off to the left side to finish off your notebook-paper nails.

FREESTYLE TIPS

• French tips don't always have to follow the natural curve of your nail. Paint on angled French tips to add a quirky edge to your mani.

TO DOWNLOAD

tinyurl.com/
hzpo5ao

Maths

School is now in session! Everyone wants to return to school with the best nails in the class, and why not celebrate the school year by creating academic-inspired nail art? Mathematical symbols make for fun decals with an educational twist.

POTENTIAL COLOURWAYS

- Mustard yellow, white, pink, orange, green, blue, red
- Red, blue, green
- Gold, red, white, purple
- Fuchsia pink, dark green, pale blue

TO SCAN
(THEN RESIZE)

TO COLOUR
(THEN RESIZE)

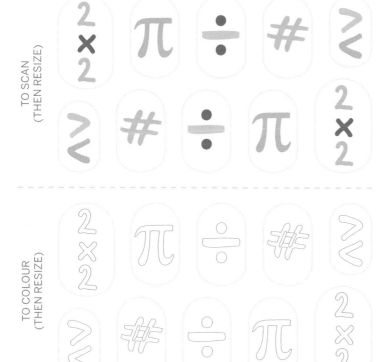

TO DOWNLOAD

tinyurl.com/
hzpo5ao

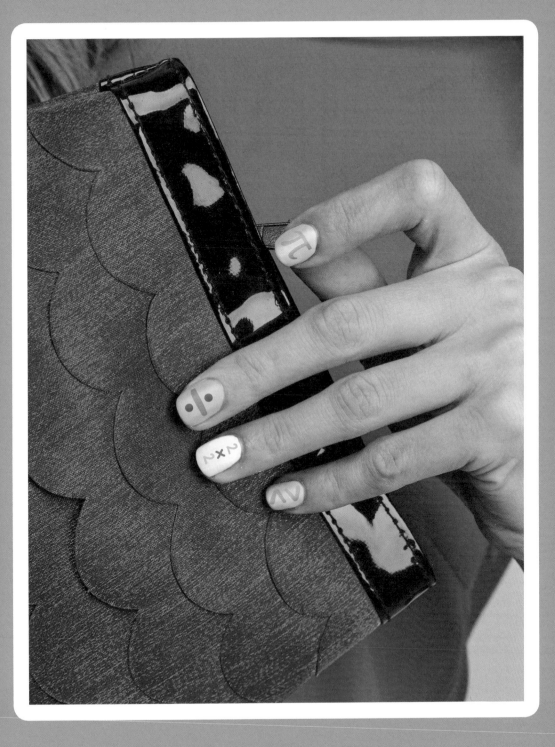

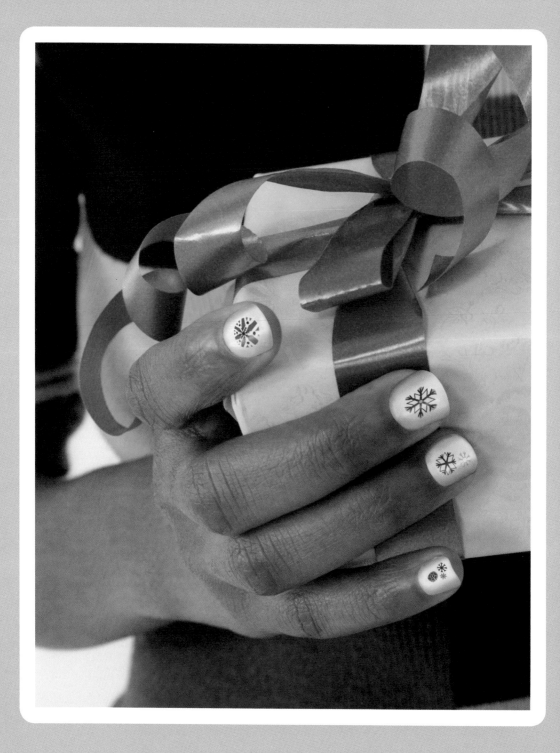

Winter

Delicate snowflakes are an enchanting emblem of the winter season. Add some sparkle with a matching accent nail in holographic or silver glitter, or embellish the snowflakes with studs or rhinestones for a flashier finish.

TO SCAN
(THEN RESIZE)

TO COLOUR
(THEN RESIZE)

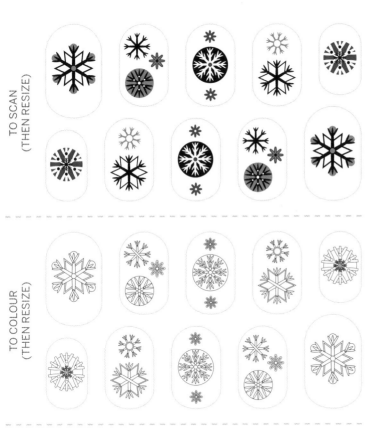

TO DOWNLOAD

tinyurl.com/
hzpo5ao

TIPS

Create a colour gradient with nail polish:

1. Apply a white base colour to the nail first, so that the colour gradient can pop.

2. Select your colours and apply each band of nail polish in turn onto a rectangular wedge make-up sponge.

3. Dab the make-up sponge onto the nail to blend the colours together.

4. Add a second thin coat of the colours if necessary.

5. Clean around the edges of the nail with nail polish remover and a cotton bud.

Autumn

Nostalgic autumn leaves signify the approach of the festive season. Leaves in warm and cosy shades of red, gold and orange will set a tranquil scene. Decorate accent nails with gold polka dots and earthy oranges.

POTENTIAL COLOURWAYS

- Red, orange, yellow, white
- Red, yellow
- Red, orange, nude
- Gold, red, yellow, orange

TO SCAN
(THEN RESIZE)

TO COLOUR
(THEN RESIZE)

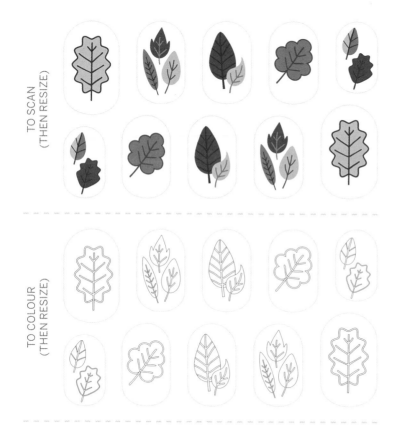

TO DOWNLOAD

tinyurl.com/
hzpo5ao

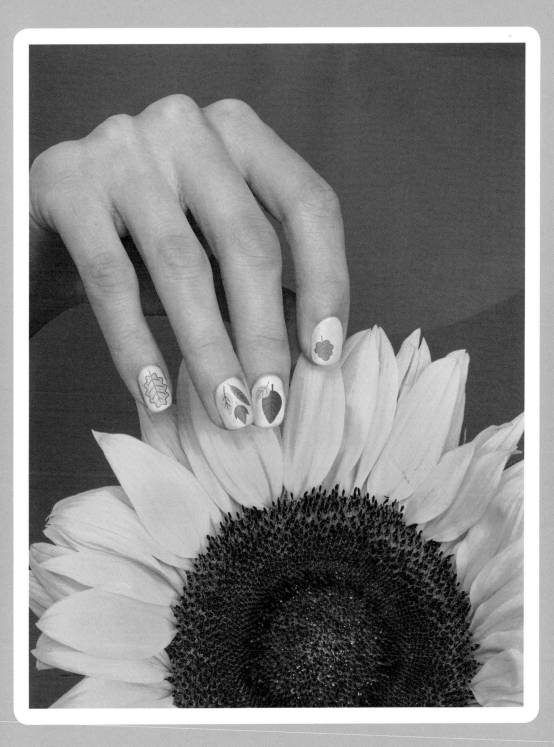

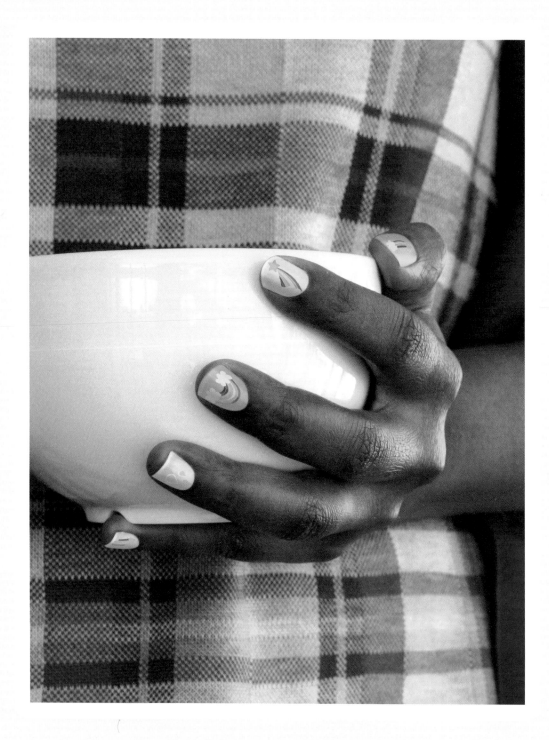

Rainbows

Pastel rainbows are sweet and whimsical motifs. Spring and summer months warrant colourful palettes, but you can soften up your manicure with candy pastels for an ethereal look.

TIPS

Paint your own cloud nails:

1. Apply a sky-blue base colour to the nail first.

2. Dip a hair grip into white nail polish. Dot this onto the nail to create puffy white clouds.

3. To make raindrops, dip a narrow nail brush in blue nail polish and add short streaks of blue below the clouds.

TO SCAN (THEN RESIZE)

TO COLOUR (THEN RESIZE)

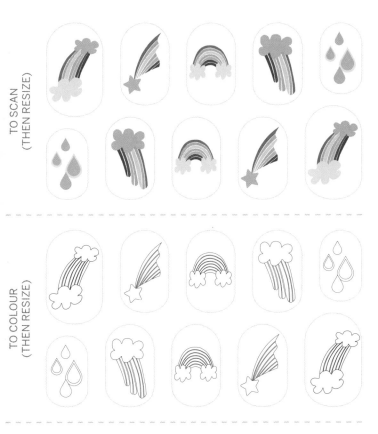

TO DOWNLOAD

tinyurl.com/ hzpo5ao

Unicorns

Infuse some light-hearted fantasy into your personal style by creating unicorn-inspired nail looks. These soft pastel decals pair well with iridescent glitter nail polish. Add extra stars and swirls and let your imagination run wild.

POTENTIAL COLOURWAYS

- White, baby pink, mint green, light lavender, light yellow, silver
- Gold, purple, pink, pale blue
- Pale blue, lilac, yellow
- Pale blue, baby pink, purple

TO SCAN (THEN RESIZE)

TO COLOUR (THEN RESIZE)

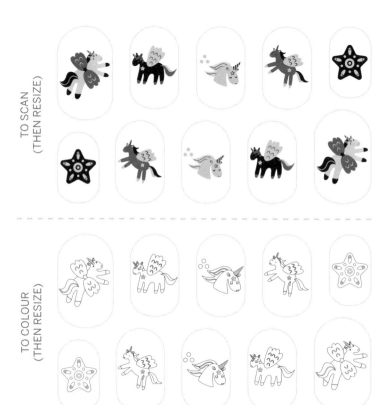

TO DOWNLOAD

tinyurl.com/ hzpo5ao

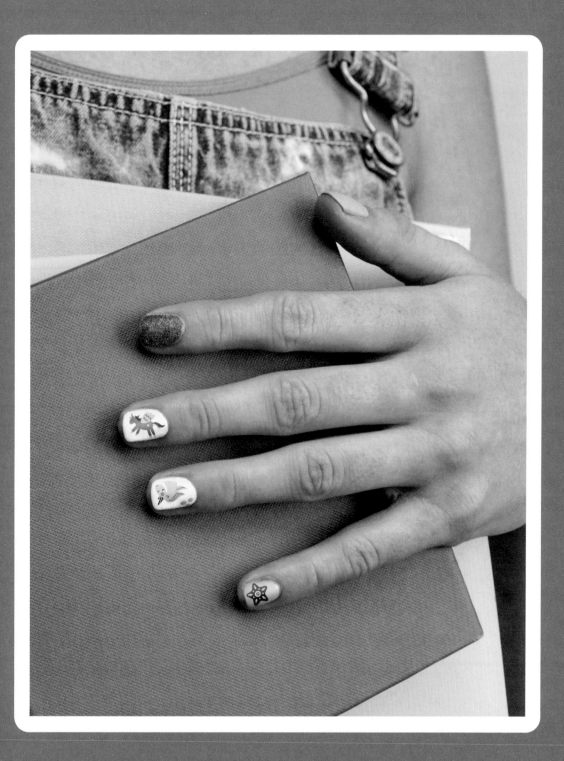

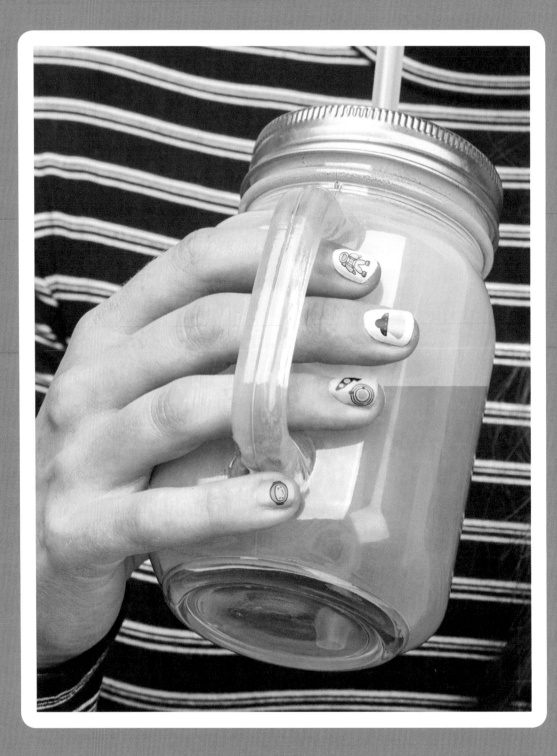

Spaceman

Fly me to the moon! Explore the stars with little moon men at your fingertips. All you need to create an interstellar look is black, purple and blue nail polish, a sponge, a toothpick and these cute decals. Add some extra glam by finishing off the look with a layer of glitter nail polish.

TO SCAN
(THEN RESIZE)

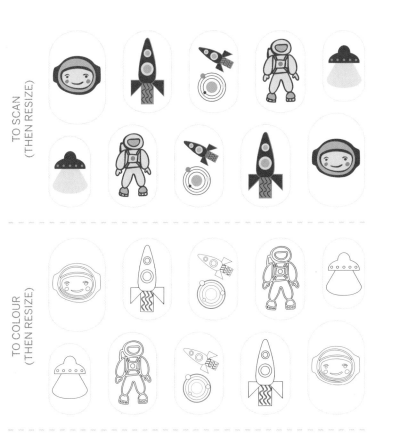

TO COLOUR
(THEN RESIZE)

TO DOWNLOAD

tinyurl.com/
hzpo5ao

Stars and Planets

Do you want nails that are out of this world? Aim high with an intergalactic look that will take your mani to the next level. Stars, colourful planets and similar astronomy themes are quirky and look beautiful with glitter accents. Or you can cover your entire nail in fine iridescent glitter nail polish for all-over space-inspired shimmer.

POTENTIAL COLOURWAYS

- Purple, blue, fuchsia pink, mint green
- Black, purple, silver
- Green, pink, purple, silver
- Teal, black, purple, gold

TO SCAN (THEN RESIZE)

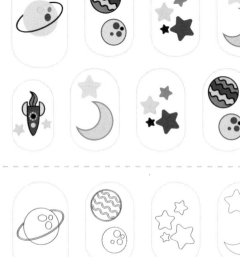

TO COLOUR (THEN RESIZE)

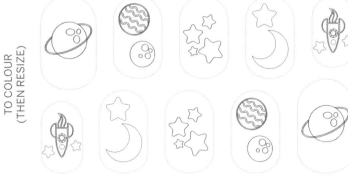

TO DOWNLOAD

tinyurl.com/ hzpo5ao

86

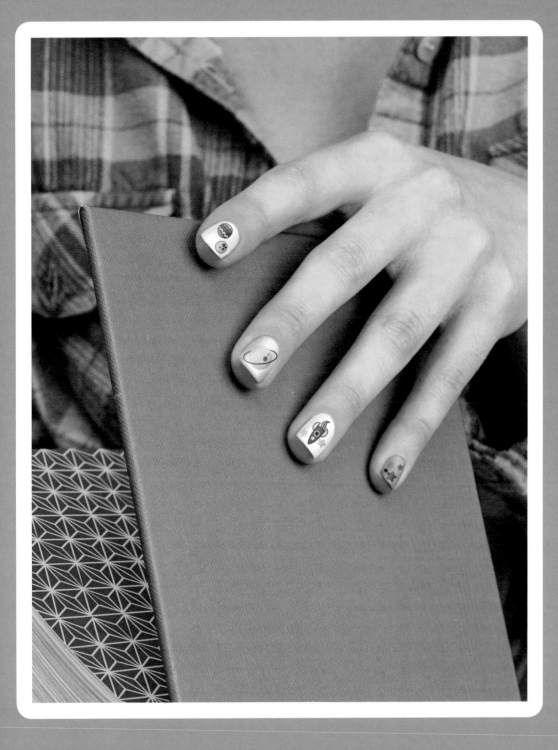

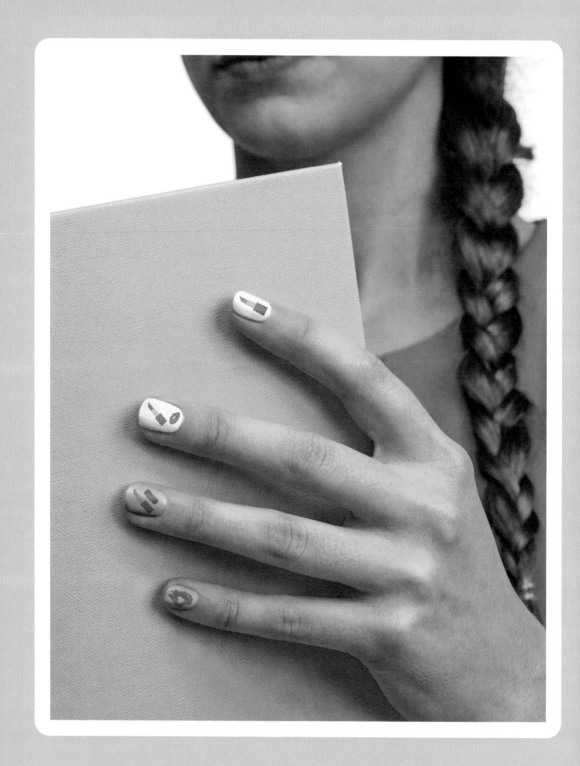

Lipstick

Beautify your nails with make-up – make-up-themed nail art, that is! Playful lipstick motifs are a fun way to celebrate your love for cosmetics. Stick with classic red and pink shades or go wild with outrageous colours. Keep the background polish neutral and let the lips do all the talking!

TIPS

Create a red lips motif on your nails:

- Paint your nails in a single contrasting shade to act as your background colour.

- Dip a toothpick in red nail polish. Draw a top lip shape by creating an elongated letter 'M'.

- Dip the toothpick in red nail polish again, and finish the mouth shape by adding a slighly curved bottom lip underneath.

TO SCAN (THEN RESIZE)

TO COLOUR (THEN RESIZE)

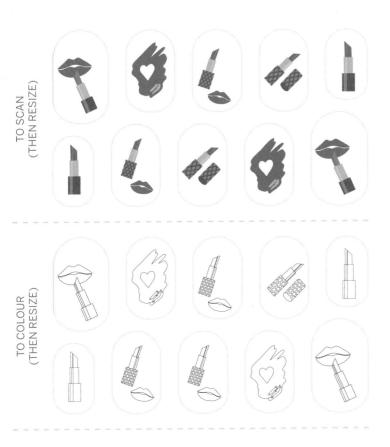

TO DOWNLOAD

tinyurl.com/ hzpo5ao

89

Nail Polish

If you love nail art, adding nail-polish bottle motifs to your nails is an obvious choice. Match your accent nails to the decal bottle shades for a colour-coordinated look, and use glitter accents for added glamour.

POTENTIAL COLOURWAYS

• Red, baby pink, white, black, silver

• Pink, blue, purple, teal

• Pale blue, turquoise, dark blue

• Red, white, pink

TO SCAN (THEN RESIZE)

TO COLOUR (THEN RESIZE)

TO DOWNLOAD

tinyurl.com/ hzpo5ao

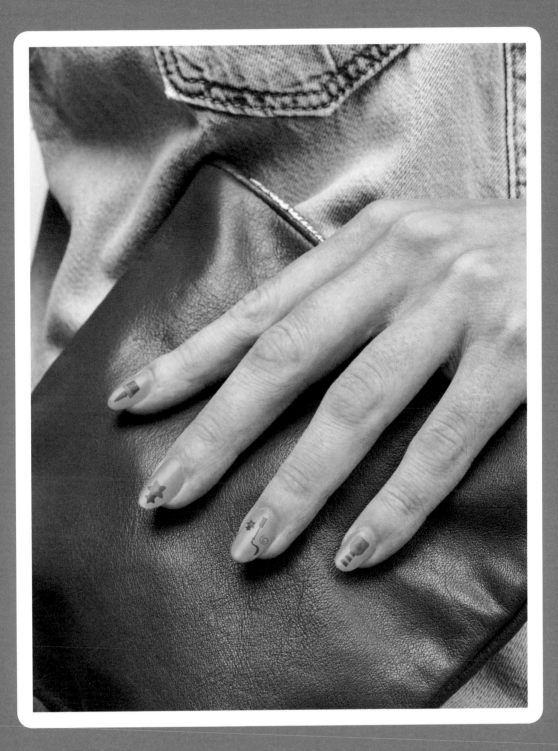

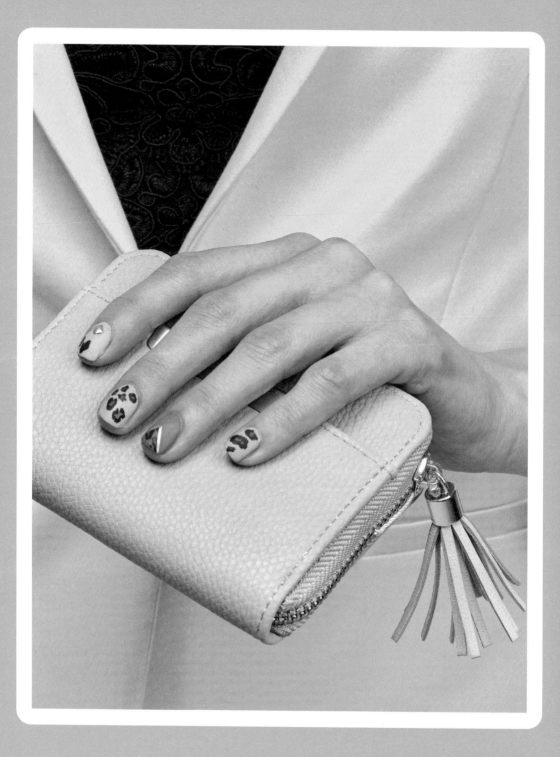

Leopard

Leopard print is widely considered to be a staple in the fashion world. Complement it with one bold colour (black, blue or red, for example) and harness the energy of the majestic leopard to wear your look with confidence. Why not create leopard-print nail tips and highlight your spots with gold metallics?

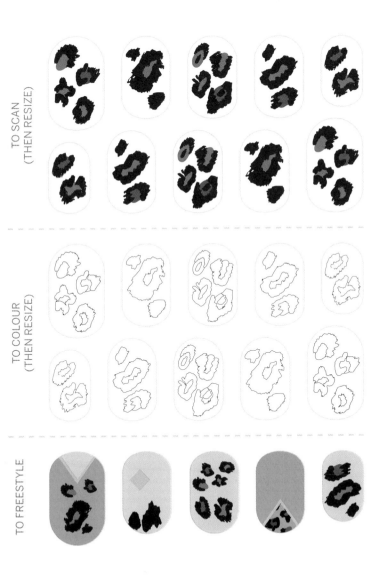

TO SCAN (THEN RESIZE)

TO COLOUR (THEN RESIZE)

TO FREESTYLE

TIPS

DIY leopard-print nail art:

1. Paint your entire nail with a gold nail polish.

2. Dip a toothpick in black nail polish. Draw a small 'c' shape. Repeat, changing the size and direction of the 'c', until the entire nail is covered; the more varied the spots are, the better the leopard print will turn out.

FREESTYLE TIPS

• You don't have to use these patterned decals across the whole of the nail. For a sharp, modern look, consider cutting them into geometric shapes, such as triangles, and applying to the tip of the nail. Paint a gold border (or use gold stickers) along two sides of the triangle to make the pattern really pop.

TO DOWNLOAD

tinyurl.com/hzpo5ao

93

Zebra

Call it the circle of life. Fashion trends are fickle, but animal prints are here to stay. Chic zebra print is a simultaneously modern and organic design that looks beautiful as an accent nail. Finish the look with polka dots in complemantary colours or shimmering metallics.

POTENTIAL COLOURWAYS

• Fuchsia pink, purple, teal, orange, white

• Yellow, green, white

• Orange, gold, green

• Black, white

TO SCAN (THEN RESIZE)

TO COLOUR (THEN RESIZE)

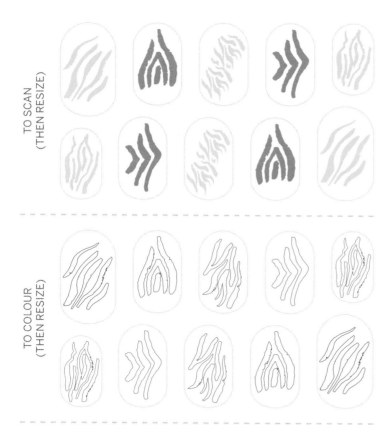

TO DOWNLOAD

tinyurl.com/ hzpo5ao

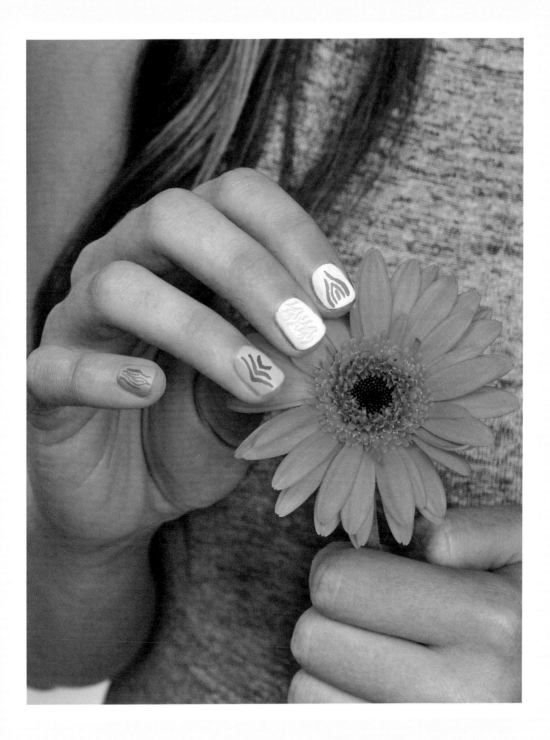

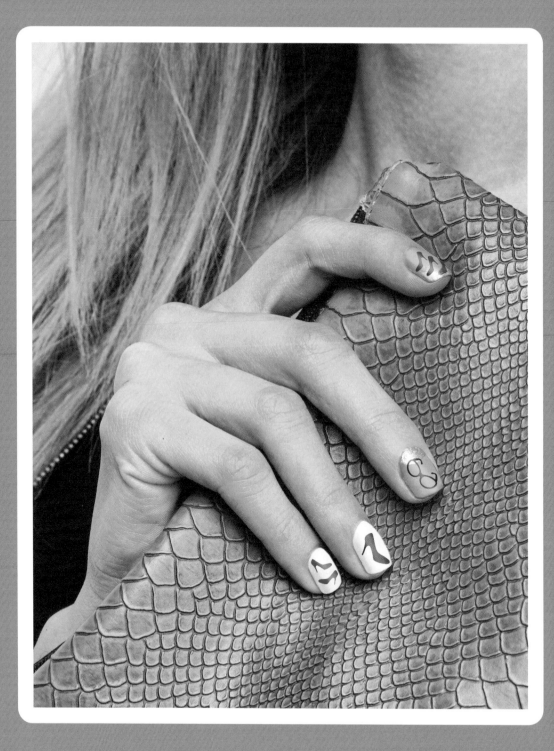

Shoes and Specs

Are you a shoe lover? The sleek lines of a stiletto heel create a classic silhouette that exudes femininity. You are never too young or too old to appreciate a great pair of heels. Bring in the glasses for added specs appeal and decorate accent nails with chic stripes and cute bows.

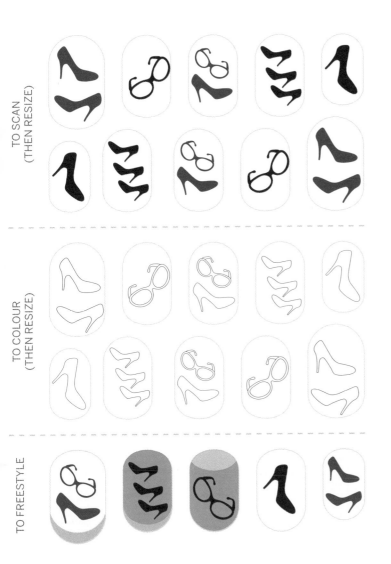

TO SCAN
(THEN RESIZE)

TO COLOUR
(THEN RESIZE)

TO FREESTYLE

TIPS

Create another fashionista accent with bow nail art:

1. Dip a hair grip into your favourite pink nail polish. Add dots to the nail in a figure-of-eight shape.

2. Form two bow ends by adding two rows of dots originating from the centre of the figure of eight.

FREESTYLE TIPS

• Add shimmer to your shoes and specs with glitter highlights. Paint half-moon shapes at the top of your nail using your favourite glitter polish, or at the tips of your nails for a super-sparkly finish.

TO DOWNLOAD

tinyurl.com/
hzpo5ao

Dresses

Celebrate your passion for fashion with dressy nail art! Nail art and fashion are forms of personal expression and together they illustrate polished style. Dress up your nails in these bows, dresses and blouses, and paint accent nails in white and pretty pastels.

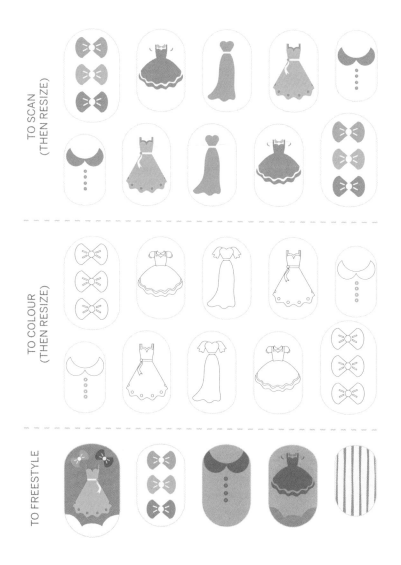

TO SCAN
(THEN RESIZE)

TO COLOUR
(THEN RESIZE)

TO FREESTYLE

POTENTIAL COLOURWAYS

- Turquoise, purple, white, pink, orange
- White, baby pink, mint green, lilac, yellow
- Pale blue, baby pink, purple
- Black, white, silver

FREESTYLE TIPS

To create pinstripes:

1. Dip a long, thin synthetic brush into purple (or colour of your choice) nail polish.
2. Wipe off any excess nail polish from the brush to prevent drips.
3. Rest your wrist on a table while holding the brush.
4. To create a steady line, apply the brush onto the nail surface and hold it still while slowly moving the nail you are painting.

TO DOWNLOAD

tinyurl.com/
hzpo5ao

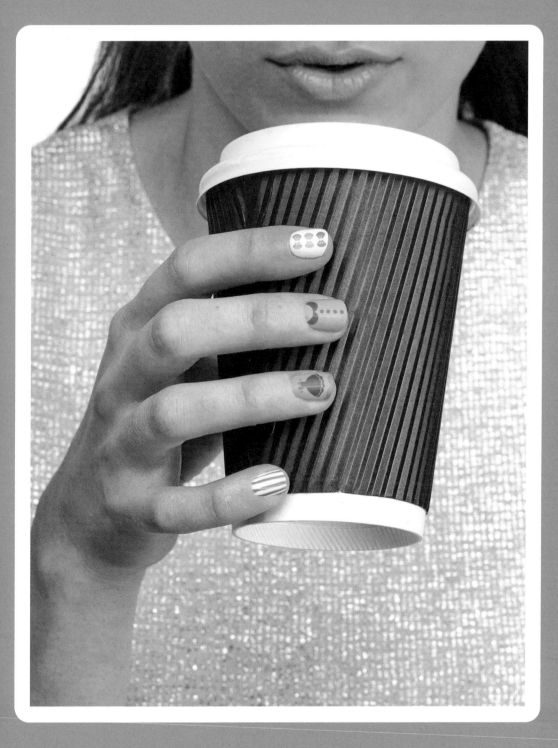

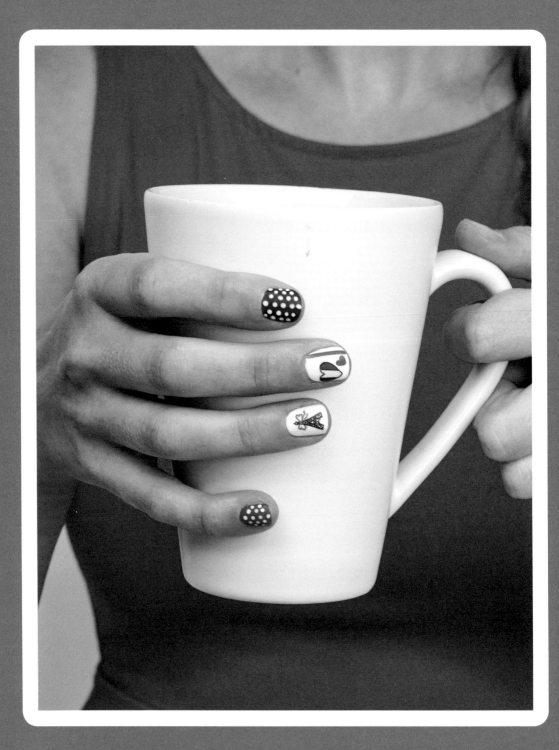

Ooh La La!

Get inspired by your dream destinations with travel-themed nail art! Take your nails on a trip to Paris with these Eiffel Tower and French flag designs. Paint accent nails in blue and red with white polka dots for a quirky, coordinated look.

TO SCAN (THEN RESIZE)

TO COLOUR (THEN RESIZE)

TO FREESTYLE

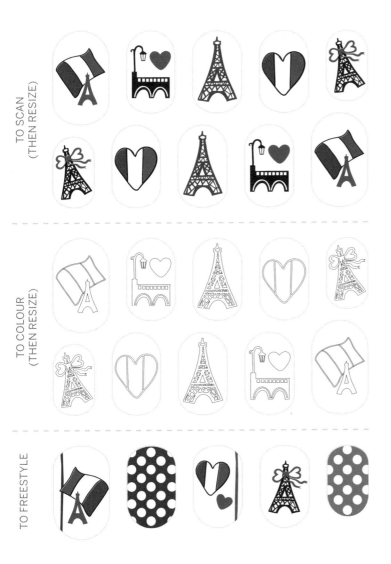

TIPS

Paint your own geometric colour-block nails:

1. Choose three contrasting colours. Use the lightest colour to paint the entire nail. Wait for each colour to dry before moving on to the next one.

2. Swipe the second-lightest colour at a diagonal to create a large triangle shape on the bottom half of the nail.

3. With the darkest colour of the three, fill in half of the triangle.

FREESTYLE TIPS

To create coordinated polka dots with French flair:

1. Apply the base colours (blue and red) to your nails.

2. Take a hair grip and dip the round end of it in white nail polish.

3. Dab the end of the hair grip onto the nail to create your polka dots.

TO DOWNLOAD

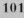

tinyurl.com/
hzpo5ao

101

Around the World

There's a whole world of nail art out there to explore! Send your nails on a summer holiday with prints inspired by maps and globes, aeroplanes and suitcases. Pair with accent nails in fresh cyan and white for a truly global appeal.

POTENTIAL COLOURWAYS

- Steel blue, light yellow, cyan, white
- Black, white, silver, purple, pale blue
- White, silver, navy blue
- Green, pale blue, dark blue
- Silver, grey, steel blue

TO SCAN
(THEN RESIZE)

TO COLOUR
(THEN RESIZE)

TO DOWNLOAD

tinyurl.com/
hzpo5ao

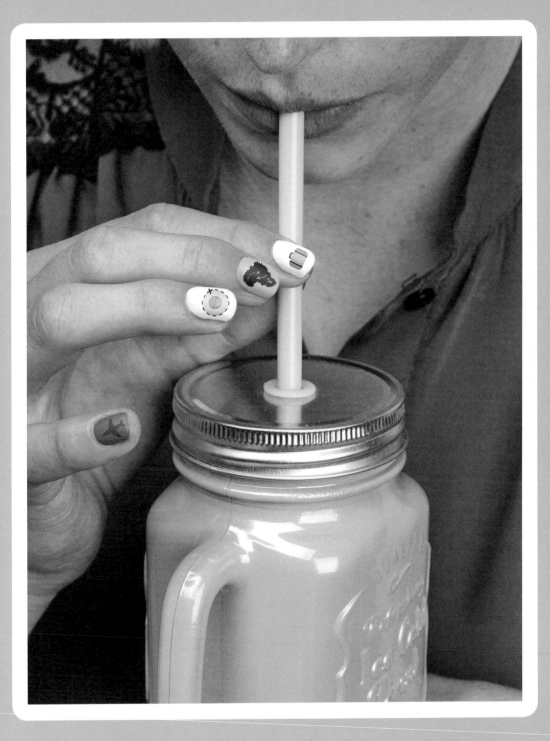

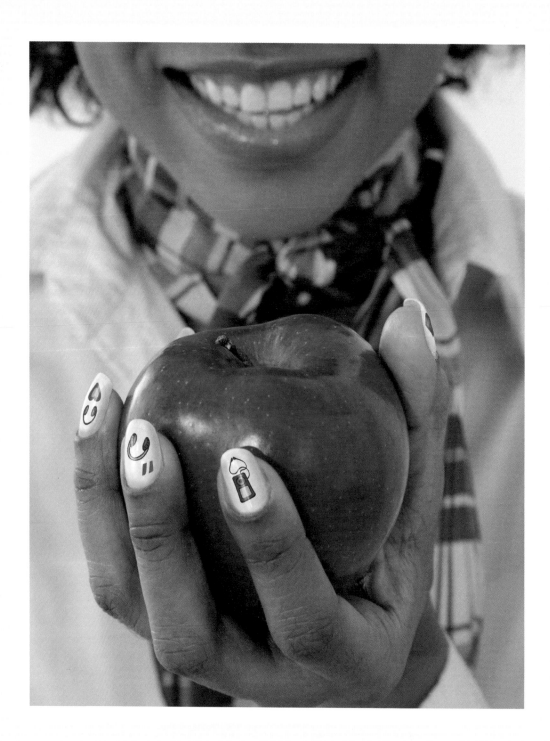

Headphones

Bring out your inner rock star and let your nails rock out with modern music-themed headphone designs. Add an extra note of quirkiness with these MP3 players and musical directions. Play up your decal designs by painting background nails with bright opaques such as orange or turquoise.

TO SCAN (THEN RESIZE)

TO COLOUR (THEN RESIZE)

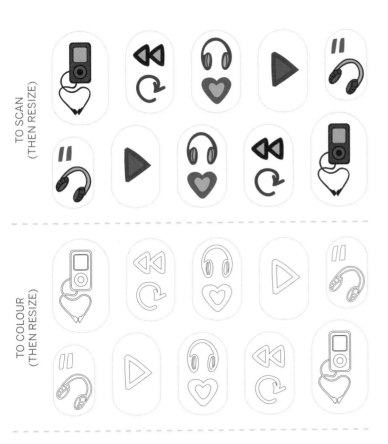

TIPS

Add some heavy metal with metal nail studs:

1. Dip a toothpick in some nail glue and apply small dots to the nails.

2. Before the glue dries, apply small metal nail studs with your tweezers.

Create a high-coverage glitter accent nail without a ton of layers:

1. Apply a matching non-glitter nail polish to the nail as your base colour.

2. Apply glitter nail polish to a wedge make-up sponge. The sponge will absorb excess clear nail polish, which will give you much thinner layers.

3. Dab the sponge onto the nail to add a thin layer of glitter. Repeat a number of times to achieve full glitter coverage.

TO DOWNLOAD

tinyurl.com/ hzpo5ao

Keys and Notes

Music is a universal language that can calm the soul. . . and make your nails look fab! Classic music designs featuring the stave, treble clef and notes will speak volumes about your passion for music. Pair with glitter accents and black polka dot designs to hit the perfect note.

POTENTIAL COLOURWAYS

- Medium orchid, blue-violet, red, white, grey
- Black, white, red
- Grey, red, black, silver
- Black, white, fuchsia pink, gold glitter

TO SCAN (THEN RESIZE)

TO COLOUR (THEN RESIZE)

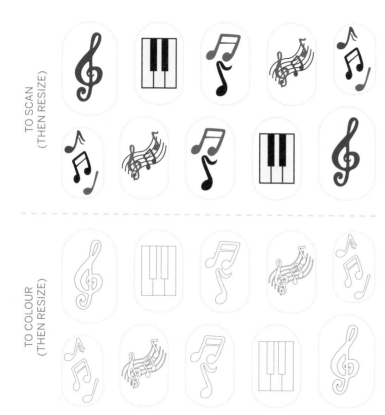

TO DOWNLOAD

tinyurl.com/ hzpo5ao

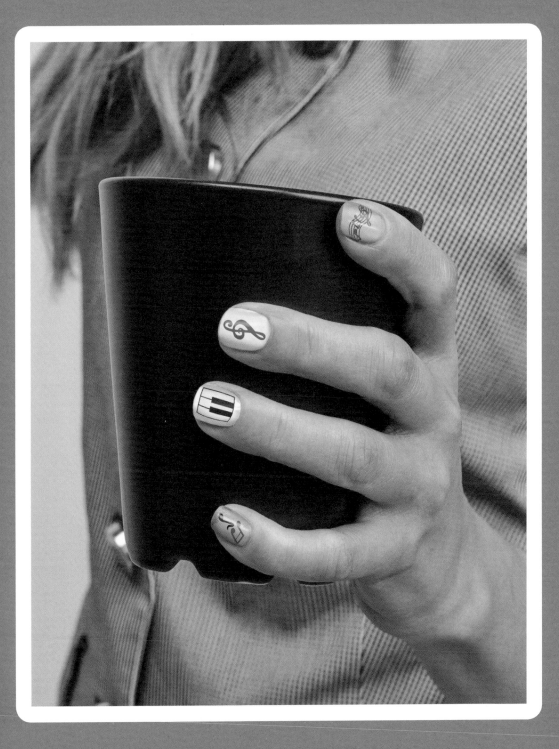

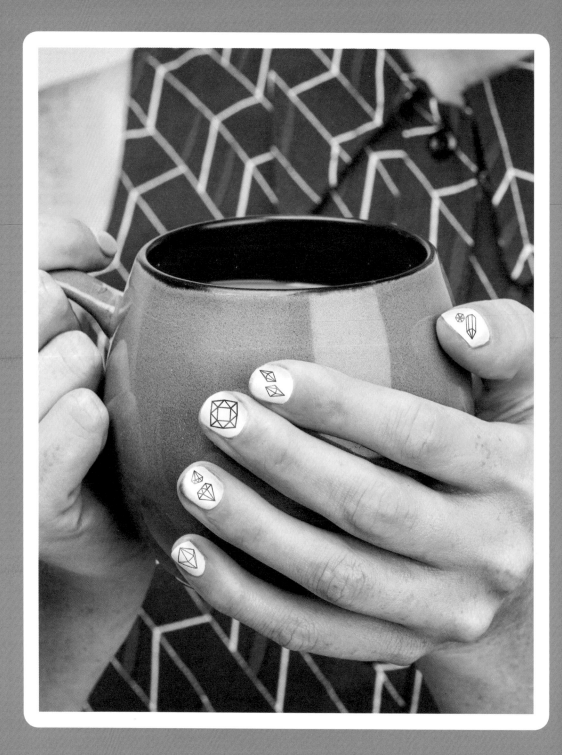

Crystal Outlines

Rock a haute hippie look! Since the time of ancient Egyptians, crystals have been seen as a form of alternative medicine. Today, crystals and natural gems are associated with boho fashion and trendy summer music festivals. Apply over marbled nails to create a gem of a mani!

TIPS

Create marbled stone nails:

1. Paint your nails white.

2. Take a small piece of cling film and scrunch it up. Dip the plastic wrap into silver polish and dab it onto your nails to emulate natural marble splotches.

3. To add lines and striations in the marble, dip a narrow brush into a dark grey nail polish and paint thin streaks across the nail.

FREESTYLE TIPS

• Add delicate French tips for a contemporary pop of colour on neutral nails.

• Remember that you don't always have to apply decals in the centre of your nail bed – geometric outlines such as these can look great positioned at the tip and cut off mid-design where they reach the edge of the nail.

TO SCAN
(THEN RESIZE)

TO COLOUR
(THEN RESIZE)

TO FREESTYLE

TO DOWNLOAD

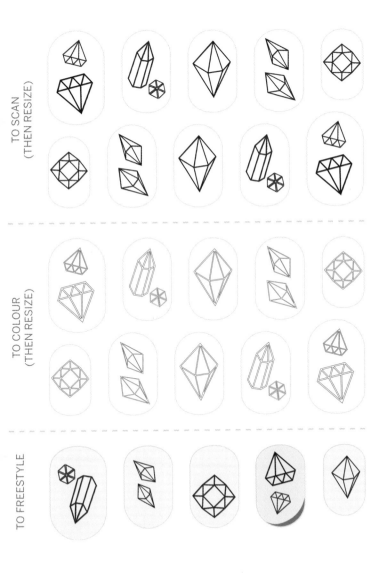

tinyurl.com/
hzpo5ao

Coloured Crystals

Colour in your crystals and gemstones with nail polish for a customized look. Get colour inspiration from birthstones and zodiac colours. Apply them over neutral colours to make your crystals pop, or paint nails in gold glitter for a look that will rock your world!

POTENTIAL COLOURWAYS

- Fuchsia pink, purple, turquoise, gold
- Pale blue, pale pink, dark blue
- Teal, silver, purple
- Navy blue, lilac, fuchsia pink, gold glitter

FREESTYLE TIPS

- You can mix and match a little with these decals. Try fitting several of the smaller crystals onto one nail, arranged as you like best, to make your designs truly unique.

TO SCAN (THEN RESIZE)

TO COLOUR (THEN RESIZE)

TO FREESTYLE

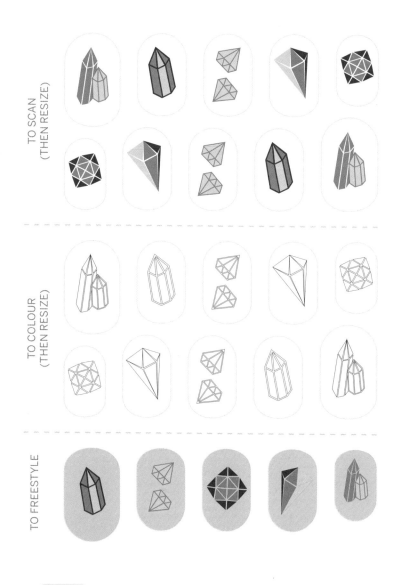

TO DOWNLOAD

tinyurl.com/ hzpo5ao

110

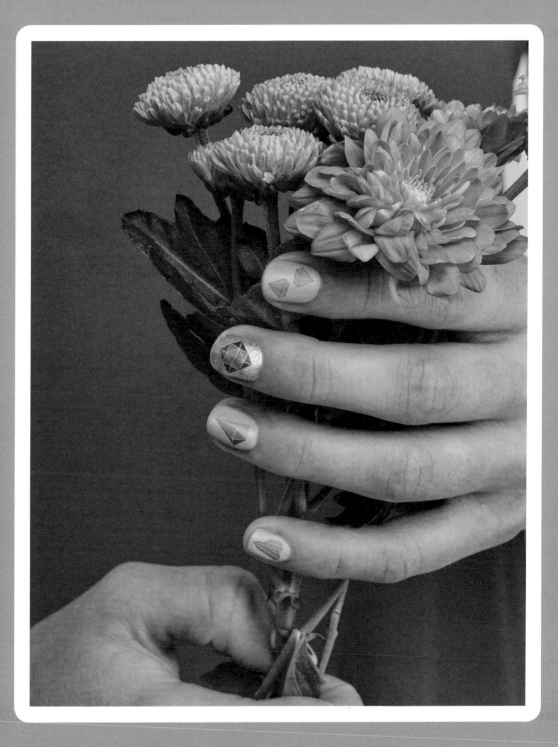

4 EMBELLISHING YOUR DECALS

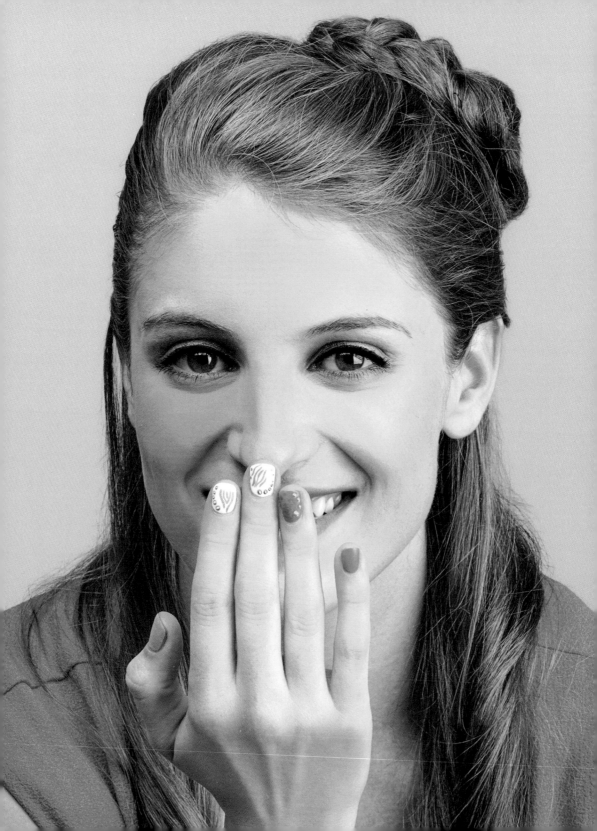

Polish

Bring blank nail decals to life by colouring them in with your own nail polish! You can completely change a look by using different colour combos, so experiment and use your colour choices to create a unique design. Customize your manicure even further by adding extra details to the decals with simple nail art designs.

YOU WILL NEED

- Nail polish colours
- Aluminium foil
- Toothpicks
- Narrow synthetic brush
- Nail polish remover
- Paper towel
- Nail topcoat

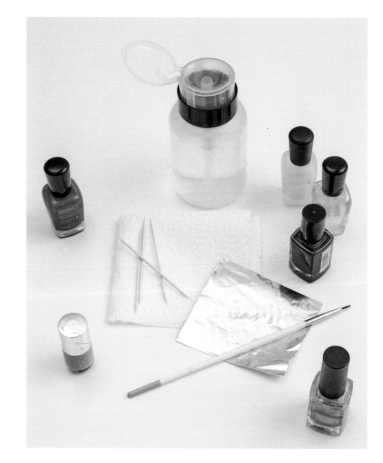

1

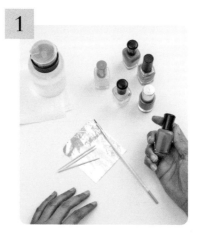

Choose your nail polish colours. You can mix existing colours together to create new shades.

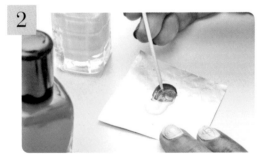

2

A piece of aluminium foil will act as your paint palette. Add drops of nail polish to your palette and mix the colours with a toothpick if necessary.

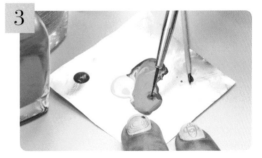

3

Dip a narrow synthetic brush into the nail polish to pick up your colour of choice.

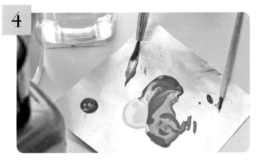

4

Wipe any excess nail polish from the brush onto the paint palette.

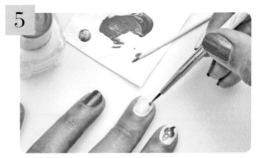

5

Add colour to the nail decal – fill in portions of the decal or add your own freehand nail art to complement the decal and create your very own masterpiece!

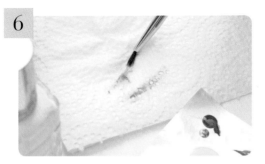

6

When you're ready to paint with a different nail colour, wipe down the synthetic brush with a bit of paper towel soaked in nail polish remover, to clean off the brush before you start on your next colour.

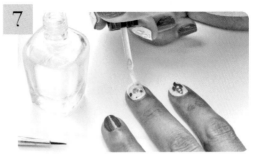

7

Once your painting is complete, add topcoat to the design to seal in the colour.

Chunky loose glitter

Add sparkle to your decals with glitter! Loose craft glitter comes in lots of colours, shapes and sizes. Try placing the glitter in a specific formation to highlight your design, or apply over the entire nail for full-on bling!

YOU WILL NEED

- Nail topcoat
- Aluminium foil
- Toothpicks
- Chunky loose glitter

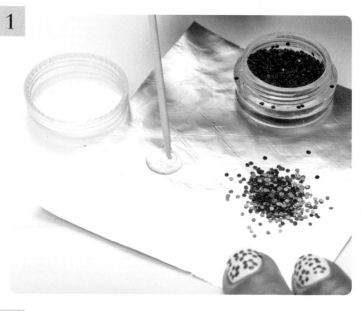

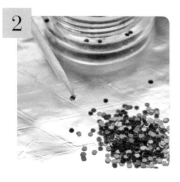

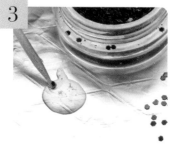

1. Add a drop of topcoat to a piece of aluminium foil. Dip the end of a toothpick into the topcoat.

2. Pick up individual pieces of glitter with the end of your toothpick.

3. Gently dip each glitter piece back into the drop of topcoat. This small amount of topcoat will help the glitter piece stick to your nail.

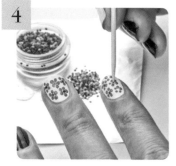

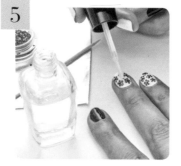

4. Apply the individual piece of glitter to the nail.

5. Repeat steps 1 to 4 to add more glitter pieces in whatever formation you like. Add another layer of topcoat to seal it in.

Fine loose glitter

Fine glitter results in a sophisticated sparkle and is particularly good for creating glitter French tips. Alternatively, use it to pick out elements of your designs to make your nail decals dazzle.

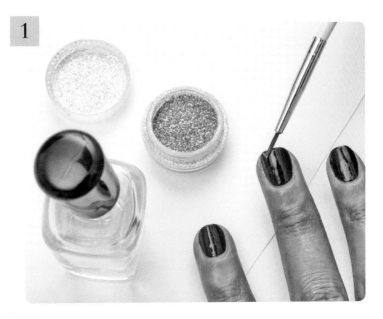

1

YOU WILL NEED

- Paper
- Nail topcoat
- Fine loose glitter
- Sticky tape

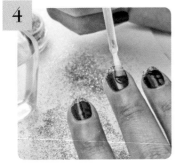

2

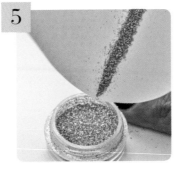

3

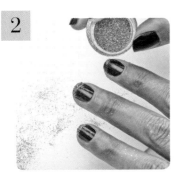

4

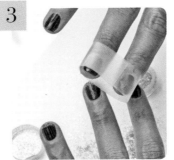

5

1. Place a piece of paper on your workspace. Apply topcoat to the part of the nail where you wish to add glitter.

2. Gently sprinkle the loose glitter over the nail, allowing the leftover glitter to fall onto the piece of paper underneath.

3. Tap off the excess from the skin and pick up any remaining glitter with a piece of sticky tape.

4. Apply topcoat to seal in the loose glitter.

5. Carefully pick up the piece of paper and funnel the extra loose glitter back into the glitter container for later use.

Studs & rhinestones

Studs and jewels are a fun and easy way to embellish your nail decals and are great for nail art beginners and pros alike. Studs can be used for metallic accents to toughen up a look, while rhinestones add an eye-catching glint to any mani. Use sparingly for subtle glimmers or cover the nail for a glamorous look to take you into evening.

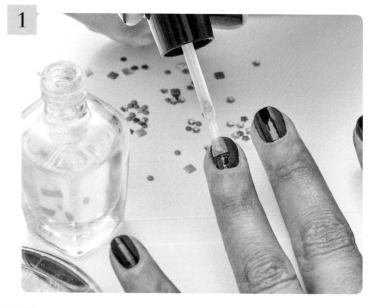

YOU WILL NEED

- Nail base coat and topcoat
- Nail glue (if needed)
- Tweezers, toothpick or wax crayon
- Studs or jewels

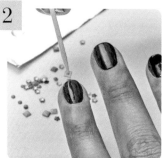

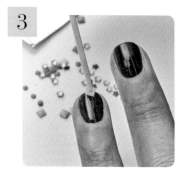

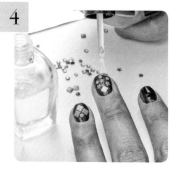

1. Add base coat to the area that you wish to embellish. For a longer-lasting hold, apply a drop of nail glue instead.

2. Use tweezers, a toothpick dipped in topcoat or the pointed end of a wax crayon to pick up each individual nail embellishment.

3. Place the nail embellishment onto the wet base coat or nail glue.

4. Add topcoat to seal in all of the decorations.

Stickers

Decorative stickers are a great way to embellish your mani – and they are so easy to use. They come in so many different colours, shapes and sizes – the possibilities are endless. Using stickers can be a really quick way to boost a plain mani, and with so many shapes and themes to choose from, there will always be a sticker to match your mood!

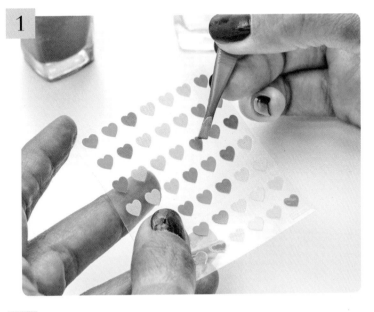

YOU WILL NEED

• Nail stickers
• Tweezers
• Topcoat

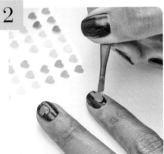

1. Start with dry, polished nails. Peel off the decorative nail stickers from their paper backing.

2. Carefully apply the nail stickers to the nails using tweezers.

3. Apply topcoat to seal in each of the nail stickers.

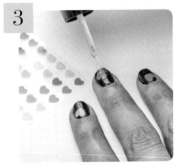

5 NAIL SPA

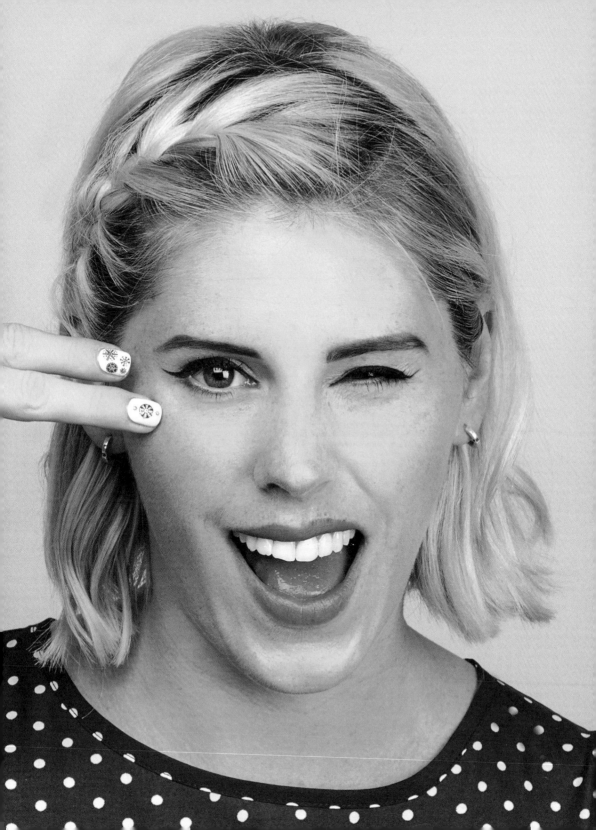

DIY mani

Follow these nail-care basics to create a beautiful manicure that really lasts.

Oil removal: Make sure your nails are clean and oil-free before applying nail polish. A completely greaseless surface is needed for nail polish to adhere and last. Strip the nails by lightly swiping them with nail polish remover. Apply remover with a piece of paper towel, since cotton balls can leave fuzz on the nail. Avoid nail polish remover products with moisturizing properties such as vitamin E, lanolin or aloe, since these will deposit oils.

Base coat: The base coat acts as a foundation that protects your natural nails and gives the polish something to adhere to. Apply a single layer of base coat to the nails and let it dry for two minutes before applying nail colour.

Clean up: If you notice any nail polish on the skin around your nail beds, dip a toothpick or wooden stick into nail polish remover and wipe away the excess nail polish from the skin.

Applying nail polish: For an even finish, apply two thin layers of nail colour. Swipe the nail polish brush down the middle of the nail. Add a swipe of colour down the left side of the nail, then the right. Avoid applying thick layers, because the nail polish can peel off your nails in sheets. Make sure you let each coat of nail polish dry for a full two minutes before adding another. This waiting time allows the nail polish solvents to evaporate fully.

Topcoat: The purpose of topcoat is to leave nail colour shiny and protected from chipping and peeling. Once the nail polish has dried fully, apply a single, even layer of topcoat to each nail.

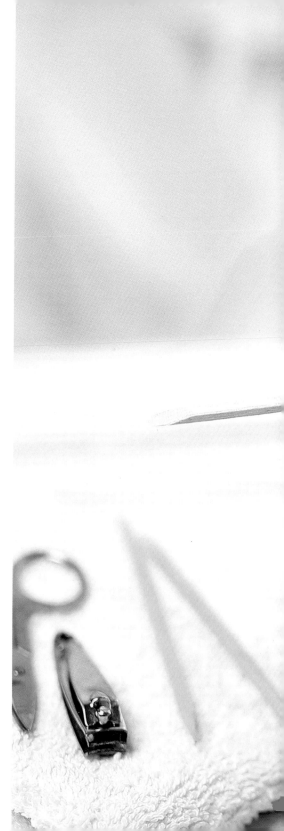

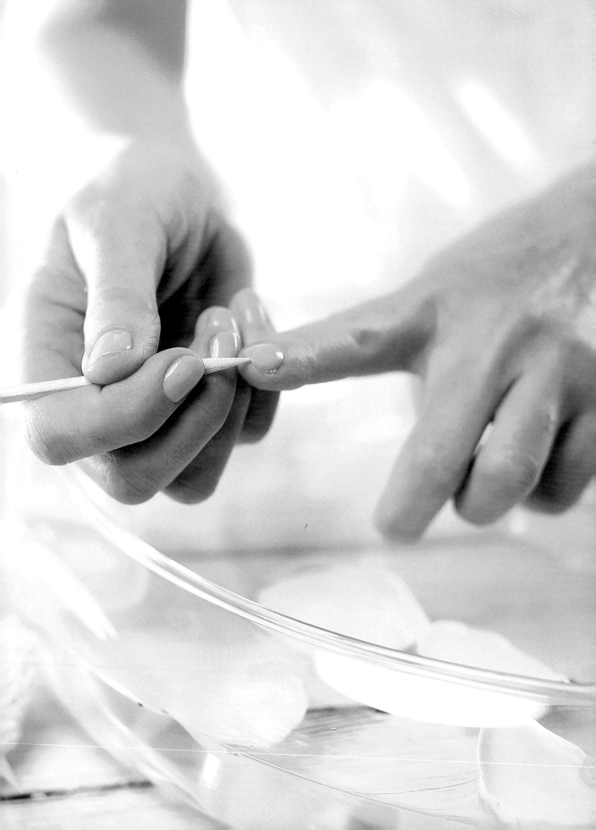

Shaping

Ready to grab a nail file and update your look? There are three common nail shapes to consider: round, square or 'squoval'. Ultimately, nail shapes and lengths will depend on your personal preference and what works with and fits into your own lifestyle.

Nail files and types: Choose an emery board or glass nail file with a fine grit. Avoid metal nail files, since they can be too hard and may damage natural nails. A nail file with a higher grit number is gentler and has a softer quality than one with a lower number. A 240-grit nail file is suitable for natural nails. Avoid filing the nails in a back-and-forth sawing motion, and only file in a single direction, from side to centre.

Round: To get rounded nails, continue to file the edges of the nail bed until you end up with a smooth half-circle. The rounded nail shape is perfect for short nails. It is the most natural shape and is very durable due to the lack of sharp edges. Nails that are slightly longer with rounded oval nail tips can elongate the fingers and make them appear elegant and feminine.

Square: A modern nail shape that works well with mid-length nails. File straight across the nail in a single direction to give the nail a squared-off shape. The square shape has a widening effect and makes your nail bed appear wider and shorter than before. Unfortunately, nail polish can chip due to the sharp corners.

'Squoval': A combination of the round and square nail shapes. This popular look is universally flattering to all nail beds. To achieve this look, file down the centre of the nail bed straight across in a single direction. Round off the sides of your nails with the nail file at a slight angle to soften the corners. With their rounded corners, squoval nails tend to chip less than square nails, and they are less prone to corner breakage since the edges are able to absorb shock.

Cuticle Care

Maintaining beautiful cuticles results in you having beautiful nails!

Cutting cuticles: You should avoid cutting your cuticles because they protect your newly forming nails from infection and fungus. Instead, gently push them back. Products with the term 'cuticle remover' in the name do not fully remove your cuticles; they soften the dead excess cuticle skin so this can be easily sloughed off. Apply cuticle softener or cuticle remover to the nails and let it sink in for a minute or two. With the cuticles softened, take a cuticle pusher and very gently push the cuticles back.

Moisturizing cuticles: Now that you have properly cared for your cuticles, it's time to moisturize! The use of nail polish remover and washing hands constantly can dry out the cuticles, so replenishing moisture is important to keep them looking gorgeous. There are specially formulated oils and balms created for moisturizing cuticles, but your favourite hand cream can also do the trick.

Glossary

Acrylic spray: Provides a permanent, protective gloss coating. Spray it over designs printed on waterslide decal paper when an inkjet printer has been used.

Base coat: Clear polish that is painted on the nail under the colour polish to ensure a smooth finish and to prevent staining of the nail. Just like topcoat, any clear nail polish can be used as a base coat.

Colour-blocked nails: Two (or more) distinct areas of colour (not blended) on a single nail. This look can be created simply by painting a stripe of a second colour to one side of the nail, across one end or down the middle. A more precise method involves using tape to protect the area that should not be covered with the second colour, painting the desired area then peeling off the tape to achieve a sharp line.

Cuticle: The crescent of toughened skin around the base of the fingernail.

Finish: Having a particular texture or appearance when the polish is dry. Some possible finishes are textured, matte, glitter, creme, gel, duochrome and holographic. A list of polish finishes can be found on page 12.

French tips: The effect achieved by painting the tip of the nail a different colour from the rest of the nail.

Gel nails: Gel polish is a product that uses clear and coloured gels for nail enhancements instead of ordinary polish. It is applied in a similar way to traditional nail polish, but each layer is cured under ultraviolet light. It gives a glossier and tougher finish, and lasts longer than ordinary polish – around two weeks.

Gradient nails: The effect achieved by blending two or more colours into one another on the nail.

Grit: A numerical measure of the coarseness of an emery board, nail file or buffer; these are the same numbers used to define sandpaper. Low numbers are the most coarse (such as 80–100 grit files), and the highest numbers are the least coarse (or softest).

Metallics: A type of polish with a finish that is high in shine and mirror-like.

Nail bed: The section of the finger where the nail plate rests.

Ombré nails: A look created by using five polishes in the same colour family. Each nail is painted a different colour, from lightest to darkest, to create a gradual change of colour.

Topcoat: Clear nail polish applied on top of your nail colour once it has fully dried. It acts as a sealant and creates a barrier between the surfaces of your nails and obstacles that can cause chipping and breaking.

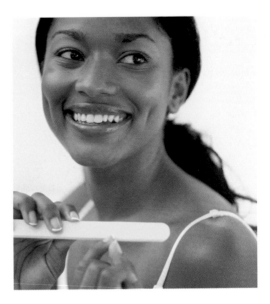

Index

Image Credits

Illustrator: Elizaveta Dmitrievna
Photographer: Neal Grundy
Nail Technician: Alex Frost
Stylist: Nicola Smith
Models: Jenny Rowlandson,
Aida Hosseini, Emily Egan,
Jaye Brown, Sienna Brown

Page 7 Shutterstock
Page 76 Getty Images
Page 104 Getty Images
Page 123 Shutterstock
Page 125 Stockbyte, Getty Images

Author biography

Janelle Estep is a self-taught nail artist and vlogger best known via her popular website and heavily subscribed YouTube™ channel 'elleandish'. By day she works as an engineer in the heart of Silicon Valley in California, where she also lives.